HYPNOTHERAPY

The Art And Science of Transformational Healing

DANIELLE AITKEN

PHP

COPYRIGHT

All characters, case examples, and descriptions in this book are presented in a fictionalised and de-identified manner. Names, identifying details, and circumstances have been changed to protect privacy. Any resemblance to actual persons, living or deceased, including clients or patients, is purely coincidental and unintentional.

Nothing in this book is intended to replace professional medical, psychological, or therapeutic advice, diagnosis, or treatment. Readers are encouraged to seek appropriate professional support for their individual needs.

The author and publisher have made every effort to credit copyright holders for material used in this book. Any person or organisation that may have been overlooked should contact the publisher.

National Library of Australia Cataloguing-in-Publication data:

HYPNOTHERAPY: The Art And Science Of Transformational Healing

- Author: Danielle Aitken
- Editor: Sue Croft
- Cover: Danielle Aitken
- Interior design: Vellum

- Print ISBN: 978-0-6488078-9-6
- E-book ISBN: 978-0-6488078-8-9

CONTENTS

Chapter One

INTRODUCTION

Welcome

If you are reading this book, it is likely that you have an inquisitive mind and a genuine interest in understanding the principles and practice of hypnotherapy. You may be seeking evidence-based approaches for personal healing or looking to enhance your ability to support others through your own therapeutic practice. Perhaps you're in pursuit of answers to questions that traditional methods have yet to resolve. Whatever your motivation, my hope is that this book provides you with practical insights, informed guidance, and a meaningful contribution to your journey in the field of healing and wellness.

In a world that can at times feel chaotic, overwhelming, and unpredictable, it is both reassuring and profound to recognise that the capacity for change, on a chemical, physical, and emotional level, already resides within you. It is a truth steeped in ancient traditions and now scientific evidence that allows me to say with certainty that a powerful human potential to interrupt old patterns and out of date habits and to create healing and wellness, is already yours.

This innate human capacity paves the way toward greater calm, clarity, and well-being. For many, this potential remains dormant for years, present yet patiently waiting beneath the surface. When it finally emerges from the depths of our inner being into our conscious awareness, it can feel like a powerful pivotal moment, a turning point that restores a sense of self-empowered inner strength and direction.

Some of you may already be well-acquainted with this truth; for others, this awareness may be yet to unfold, or perhaps it awaits discovery within the pages of this book.

Wherever you find yourself on your personal or professional journey, whether you're seeking meaningful change in your own life, looking to deepen your therapeutic practice, or simply curious about how hypnotherapy can help unlock your inner potential, this book is here to support and guide you.

Well-structured hypnotherapy may offer a powerful pathway to personal discovery. A transformative process that invites you to explore the deeper layers of your subconscious mind. Through this exploration, you can begin to gently reshape long-standing patterns and habits that may no longer serve you. By embracing the possibility of change, you can open the door to accessing the vast, often untapped potential that exists within you.

My own journey has not been without its challenges. There was a time when my health declined so significantly that I could no longer walk or function in any familiar way. Persistent, widespread pain and intense inflammation affected every joint in my body. Even the simplest tasks were beyond my ability. However, through persistence, deep inner work, and the principles shared throughout this book, my body healed. I now recognise my own experience as a gift. An extraordinary lesson that has shaped the way I now guide others. It's from this place of lived understanding that I educate my clients to access their own innate capacity for transformation and healing.

As a clinical hypnotherapist and counsellor, I've had the privilege of witnessing incredible stories of resilience and healing, just like my own. Time and time again, I've been reminded of one universal truth: we are all capable of extraordinary healing, change and growth. Throughout the pages of this book, I invite you to get curious and explore these concepts and in doing so perhaps discover, or indeed rediscover that capability for yourself.

This book is intended to demystify hypnotherapy and provide you with practical advice, inspiring case studies and insights from the latest research and neuroscientific evidence surrounding this fascinating therapeutic approach. Whether you're seeking to become a more competent practitioner, overcome a specific challenge, strengthen your confidence, or simply reconnect with your authentic self, hypnotherapy offers a path forward.

As you read on, I encourage you to approach this work with an open heart and a curious mind. Be gentle with yourself – change often takes time, but with each step forward, you'll move closer to the life you aspire to create.

Together, let's take that first step.

Regards

Danielle Aitken

Chapter Two

HYPNOSIS: WHAT YOU MAY NOT KNOW

Before delving into any topic, it's essential to begin with a clear definition. So, what exactly is hypnosis? Interestingly, this question has long been a subject of debate, even among leading experts in the field. Despite decades of research and practice, a single, universally accepted definition of hypnosis has remained elusive, adding to the intrigue that surrounds hypnosis in the therapeutic world.

Milton Erickson an American psychiatrist and physician who is widely regarded as having been one of the most influential figures in the field of hypnotherapy described hypnosis *as a state of* ***consciousness*** *or* ***awareness*** *in which there is a marked receptiveness to ideas and understandings and an increased willingness to respond either positively or negatively to those ideas.*

Right from the outset therefore, we note a discrepancy that is to be found in many hypnosis definitions. For clarity, it may actually be easier to state what hypnosis is not. In his definition Erickson importantly states that hypnosis is *a state of consciousness : not unconsciousness or sleep.* Erickson's opinion on this, being that he was an American medical doctor, psychiatrist and neurologist specialising in medical hypnosis, touted to be the father of modern hypnosis, is therefore well worthy of our serious consideration on this specific point.

Personally, coming from my own background in the mainstream medical arena, as a Registered Nurse and Registered Midwife, I can also tell you emphatically that if your client is unconscious in a standard hypnotherapy consultation, then there is something seriously concerning going on, and you might like to call an ambulance immediately.

We are just getting started and already I hope you have learned something very important. **Hypnosis is a conscious, waking state**.

Let's look a little further at this fascinating topic. I'm sure we can all remember our first, sadly, most often completely misinformed musings about what this mysterious practice was.

As a therapist I find it interesting and sometimes frustrating to see people's responses to hearing I am a hypnotherapist. Some are fascinated, others ask if I use a swinging pocket watch or a crystal glinting in dim light, while I whisper in a lowered voice "You're getting sleepy." Others ask the almost inevitable question prompted by one too many stage show presentations, "will I cluck like a chicken?" As a serious therapist my response to this is always "only if you really want to."

When describing what a hypnotherapist is we can, once again, gain clarity from looking at what a hypnotherapist is not. Although stage hypnosis may be very entertaining, it is far removed from the reality of what hypnotherapy is and how it can be used to facilitate profound change that has the potential to transform lives. The key word here is 'therapy'. As a Hypno*therapist* I do not entertain, I do no stage shows, rather I conduct therapy by utilising the state of hypnosis. Hypnosis is a vehicle that can be utilised for taking a person on a journey from point A to point B, however as I'm sure you are very aware you may travel from point A to point B in various ways.

This leads me to my next important point. In a state of hypnosis, when as we have ascertained you are certainly *not* unconscious, you are in a heightened state of **awareness and focused attention**, and importantly you are in complete control.

What this means is that I, or even the great Milton Erickson, could never make you do anything you do not want to do, or something that is against your values or morals, no matter what the latest movie tries to tell you. So why do people in stage shows get up on stage and act in ways that are often embarrassing? The answer is simple. They choose to do so.

At its core, hypnosis is a natural state of focused attention which promotes heightened suggestibility. There are specific reasons for this heightened suggestibility, and this will be discussed in my chapter on the Brain in Hypnosis.

However, for now you may remember an experience of your own when focused attention has often led to predictable outcomes. Most people have experienced this. Think about the last time you became so engrossed in a great book or a really interesting movie that you lost touch with reality as the outside world just seemed to disappear. At the time you would not have even noticed, until someone entered your space to talk to you, and you realise you didn't hear a word they said, because you were so focused on what you were looking at or doing. Your body was still present in the room working on auto pilot, while your mind was far, far away fully immersed in some other reality. That, in essence, is a hypnotic state.

You may also have experienced this type of natural trance-like state whilst driving your car, when your mind may have been thinking about work or planning your next wonderful holiday, and you hadn't even noticed that you had gone right past your turn off some time ago. It may be a little unsettling to realise that your subconscious mind can drive that car far better than your conscious mind ever could.

Often the next common misconception surrounding hypnosis is that it is always achieved in a state of deep relaxation. Now, although in the therapy room this is often the case, it should be noted that sometimes periods of extreme stress are wonderful precipitators of being able to rapidly induce someone into trance. This can often be seen at times of emergency when a quick-thinking practitioner of hypnotherapy can calm an accident victim or someone in extreme panic, by being the most confident person on the scene, and the one to quickly take control. As a midwife I often noted this phenomenon even before I became a hypnotherapist. Some may call this a rapid induction, no relaxation needed, just a firm assertive voice, directing and convincing the patient that you are in charge, and you've got this.

Hypnotherapy can also be very effectively administered in a completely waking state. Waking hypnosis or conversational hypnosis is a skill, and one of my favourite definitions by Dr. Steve Bierman is that hypnosis is achieved from '*well-constructed language leading to, ideas evoking responses.*'

Hypnosis is not magic, nor is it mind control, or surrendering your power to someone else. On the contrary, hypnosis is about reclaiming your power and tapping into your enormous reservoir of human potential, by accessing your *sub*conscious mind to create positive change. Again, I stress, your subconscious mind is not an unconscious mind. These are very different things. In fact, it is only since the early 1990's that we have been able to observe the functioning brain in real time, using Functional Magnetic Resonance Imaging (fMRI), that we can now actually observe the physical changes that occur in the conscious brain during the state of hypnosis. It is because of this ability to observe the conscious working brain that we have been able to learn more about the brain in the last 30 years than we had learned in the preceding 200 years and we have certainly learned so much about the wonderful state of hypnosis during this time.

I will discuss what we have learned in chapter 6: *The Brain in Trance: The Neuroscience of Hypnotherapy.*

To further understand what hypnosis is, we must also understand how our minds function. Whilst intimately connected to the brain, the mind extends beyond the physical structures of the brain to encompass more subjective processes such as thought, imagination, self-awareness, problem-solving, creativity, emotional responses, memory formation and decision making to name just a few functions.

In hypnotherapy we acknowledge that the mind is comprised of two primary components: the conscious mind and the subconscious mind.

The conscious mind is the analytical mind. It is the realm of logic, evaluation, problem solving, reasoning, and willpower. It's our planning mind, where we think, make decisions and review information. However, it's also where doubt, fear, and resistance can reside. Interestingly, we often believe we are using our conscious reasoning to plan our way through life, however the conscious mind is estimated to be only approximately 7% of what we do.

The remaining 93% of functioning is therefore the subconscious mind. A vast reservoir of thoughts, feelings, survival responses, belief systems, memories and more that operate beneath our conscious awareness. It is the subconscious mind that governs our habits, automatic behaviours, and emotional responses.

For example, In the morning when you get out of bed and place your feet to the floor and walk, one foot in front of the other to the bathroom without conscious thought or automatically tie your shoelaces or even jump in your car and drive, all without thinking, you are operating on "autopilot" and your subconscious mind is in charge. This part of your mind is incredibly powerful, but it's also very suggestible. It is somewhat like a fertile garden that grows no matter what seeds are planted, a garden where even weeds will flourish. It is therefore important to be very aware that the powerful subconscious mind will respond to every thought you have without judgement, whether they're empowering beliefs or limiting ones, whether they are truths or falsities based on fertile imagination.

Hypnosis has the ability to bridge the gap between the conscious and subconscious mind. The conscious mind, due to its capacity for judgement, will often filter out ideas that challenge our pre-existing beliefs. This can make change very difficult in traditional therapeutic environments. However, through focused awareness arising from a hypnotic state, the conscious mind will generally quieten down allowing access to the subconscious mind, and if you are looking for magic this is where meaningful, lasting change can occur. Hypnosis works because of this. The bypassing of the critical analytical conscious mind allows for direct communication with the powerful subconscious, where our habits, beliefs, emotions and memories are generally stored. This process allows for new perspectives to be explored and to take root.

For instance, someone who has a fear of heights may consciously wish to overcome their anxiety, but their subconscious might be holding onto a painful or frightening memory from childhood. Hypnosis can assist the individual in reframing that memory. Because hypnosis is an experiential process, it allows the person to safely imagine and confront the previously anxiety-inducing situation whilst feeling calm and connected to their inner resources. As a result, the brain can start to reprocess the experience as safe. This ability to imagine facing the fear in a relaxed state conveys a strong message to the brain that the situation is not dangerous, enabling it to develop a new response. Ultimately, the old fear can be replaced with a sense of newfound confidence and self-empowerment.

So, what does it feel like to be in hypnosis?

Many of my clients are pleasantly surprised to find that hypnosis feels relatively normal. Contrary to popular belief, you really are in complete control in hypnosis. You can move your body, scratch your nose or even walk around the room if you so choose.

In a therapeutic setting hypnosis is often facilitated by getting clients into a deeply relaxed state where they can begin to forget the business of the world around and focus their attention inwardly. As we recall from earlier, relaxation is not hypnosis, however it can certainly be very helpful in creating an environment for a state of hypnosis to be easily achieved and particularly effective if the client is presenting in an anxious state. In the clinic relaxation is therefore commonly utilised to assist in achieving a Hypnotic Induction.

Many people describe hypnosis as a similar feeling to the moments just before you fall asleep or just as you are waking. It is true to say that every one of us who have ever fallen asleep or woken up has experienced the brain waves that correlate to the state of hypnosis. This point really debunks the theory that not everyone can be hypnotised, which we will discuss further in the next chapter *Debunking Myths About Hypnosis once and for all.*

During hypnosis some may describe their body as feeling comfortably heavy where they can't be bothered moving at all, others describe it as feeling light as a feather, and others still feel something else completely. There really is no right or wrong. Your hypnosis session will be experienced in a way that is right for you in that moment. It will unfold for you exactly as it is meant to. No two sessions are the same, just as no two people are the same. One common feature that most people will experience is that the mind becomes calm and focused. You will become less aware of your external environment and far more aware of your internal environment, but you are always in control.

Another important point is that no one can be hypnotised against their will. Hypnosis is a collaborative process, requiring your willingness and participation. A hypnotherapist acts as a facilitator and guide, but you are the one steering the ship. If a suggestion doesn't align with your values or goals, your subconscious will reject it. This is why hypnosis is so empowering. It is a collaborative active process that you participate in. It is not a process that is done *to* you, rather It is a process that is done *with* you.

So, can all people be Hypnotised? The short answer is yes.

I have sometimes had clients come to me stating that they have been told by another therapist that they cannot be hypnotised. This is not true.

Although it can be said that some people are more hypnotisable than others, any person who desires to be hypnotised, can be. Desire is the key, and like any skill, it can be cultivated with practice.

People often come to the hypnotherapy clinic as a last resort after trying many other therapeutic modalities, and it is not uncommon for hypnotherapy to succeed where other therapies have not. So, why does hypnosis often work when other therapies have failed? The answer lies in its ability to address the root cause of an issue rather than just its symptoms. By addressing the underlying beliefs and emotional drivers of those behaviours, hypnosis can uncover the subconscious triggers for the problem including self-sabotaging behaviours. In hypnotherapy these can be identified and replaced with healthier client oriented and solution focused thoughts and behaviours.

This is why hypnosis is such a powerful tool for personal transformation. Whether you're seeking to break a habit, overcome a fear, or achieve a goal, hypnosis can help you align your subconscious mind with your conscious desires, creating the momentum to follow a new direction with a sense of harmony and purpose.

Hypnotherapy is generally not a one session- quick fix, nor is it magic. So, if you come to hypnotherapy expecting and believing that you are a passive participant, and someone else will be doing the work, you are mistaken. Hypnotherapy is a goal driven, well-structured therapeutic process that requires active engagement, openness, and a willingness to explore the corridors of your own mind. For those who do choose to embark on this journey, the rewards can often be life changing.

As a hypnotherapist, I've witnessed countless moments of magnificent transformation born through a willingness to explore the possibilities this therapy has to offer. A nervous speaker stepping onto a stage with newfound confidence, clients letting go of a lifetime of self-doubt, physical manifestations, such as tics or stutters simply disappearing once the underlying emotional driver has been uncovered, smokers taking their first breath of freedom as they step toward health, and so many more. These moments remind me of the incredible resilience and potential that we each possess as human beings. Potential, achieved through accessing the magnificence of the mind – body connection that we all possess.

We began this chapter by asking the question What is hypnosis and by acknowledging that a single definition is yet to be agreed upon as we explored the great Milton Erickson's definition of hypnosis. We also acknowledged Dr. Steve Bierman's thoughts, that hypnosis is achieved from well-constructed language leading to "Ideas Evoking Responses."

I think we can confidently say that we now may be getting much closer to a concise definition regarding this previously abstract concept, as we continue to learn more about the brain in the state of hypnosis with the assistance of brain imaging. We will discuss these discoveries as we continue through the book, but for now let's look at some other definitions.

The Mayo Clinic- the largest integrated not-for-profit medical group in the world defines hypnosis as '*a changed waking state of awareness and increased relaxation that allows for improved focus and concentration.'*

The Cleveland Clinic - n the United States describes hypnosis as '*a heightened state of concentration and focused attention allowing, you to be more open to suggestions about making healthful changes in your perceptions, sensations, emotions, memories, thoughts or behaviours'*.

Dr. Michael Yapko - renowned internationally recognised authority on advanced clinical applications of hypnosis, defines hypnosis as follows:

"Hypnosis is a focused experience of attentional absorption that invites people to respond experientially on multiple levels in order to amplify and utilise their personal resources in a goal directed fashion.

When employed in the clinical context, hypnosis involves paying greater attention to the essential skills of using words and gestures in particular ways to achieve specific therapeutic outcomes, acknowledging and utilising the many complex personal, interpersonal, and contextual factors that combine in varying degrees to influence client responsiveness."

If I may humbly add my own definition to this list, I would say:

Danielle Aitken - *"Hypnosis is a natural state of altered consciousness, characterised by heightened awareness combined with an increased focus of attention which is often, but not always, facilitated by voluntary relaxation. In this state people generally experience increased suggestibility to agreeable, well-constructed language in the form of therapeutically applied suggestions utilised to bypass the critical conscious mind."*

If I were to add to this definition in light of what we now know to be true, I would also say that *"It is a state associated with very specific, identifiable changes in brain activity, observable on fMRI imaging"*

I think it is fair to say that despite the many definitions, we can all agree that hypnosis is about uncovering your existing potential, skills and resources that may be lying dormant just waiting to be discovered and all it takes is the courage to really get curious and look within. Trusting in the process, you might just find the answers you've been searching for are just beneath the surface.

Throughout this chapter, I hope I have been able to give you a better understanding of what hypnosis is, and importantly what it is not, which we go on to discuss further as we proceed throughout the book.

Chapter Three

DEBUNKING MYTHS ABOUT HYPNOSIS

There's a common misconception that hypnosis can make you do things against your will, like rob a bank, stand on a table and sing the latest 'number one hit' or dare I say it, the age-old favourite - walk like a chicken.

Therefore, to fully understand hypnosis, and hypnotherapy, we must first dispel these and other myths surrounding it.

Despite hypnotherapy's growing acceptance and recognition as a powerful therapeutic modality, in many circles hypnosis remains shrouded in myths and misconceptions. In the modern era we have access to an expanding body of science and evidence in the form of well-constructed research at our disposal, yet still there are common misconceptions that prevail.

To be completely honest, I'm not exactly sure why this is so. Perhaps when we look closely at its origins, as we will in the next chapter, we can begin to make sense of this quandary. What we do know is stage shows and movies have unfortunately done little to dispel the abundance of misinformation that continues to surround hypnosis, and in many instances, they add to it.

My aim is to debunk these misconceptions and in doing so shed light on this empowering therapeutic modality. I seek to illuminate the potential of hypnotherapy when conducted skilfully by well trained, regulated practitioners who use evidence-based practices formulated on the principles of science and research.

This chapter will address the most common myths surrounding hypnotherapy, demystifying the practice and clarifying its purpose.

What better place to start than by clearly addressing Myth 1.

Myth 1: Hypnosis Is Mind Control.

One of the most pervasive myths about hypnosis is the belief that the hypnotherapist is in control of the client and has an ability to make the client do things against their will.

As mentioned above, might I say again, I'm sure we have all seen *that* movie or *that* stage show. You know the one, where the client or participant behave in outlandish or embarrassing ways and appear to be at the mercy of the whim of the hypnotist.

Please note my deliberate use of the word hypnotist here, not hypnotherapist, as there is no therapy going on in these situations. A clinical hypnotherapist will always act in respectful, ethical ways and would never aim to embarrass or control the client.

The Truth: Hypnosis is not mind control.

The client will always retain full control over their thoughts, actions, and decisions, on stage or in the therapy room. A hypnotist or a hypnotherapist, no matter how skilled cannot force anyone to do or say anything that is against their will, values or beliefs. In reality, hypnosis actually enhances your ability to be in control. We know this because there are certain changes in brain functioning that occur when in a hypnotic state. These physiological changes allow for a state of heightened awareness and focused attention to be achieved, facilitating the client's ability to step into their full potential to embrace therapeutic tools in order to create healthy choices, overcome fears, and shift negative or outdated thoughts, feelings and behaviours.

Hypnotherapy's collaborative nature ensures best outcomes are obtained when the client actively and willingly participates in the process, whilst voluntarily embracing suggestions that are in alignment with their personal goals.

Myth 2: Hypnosis is a state of Unconsciousness.

Another common misconception, as discussed in a previous chapter is that hypnosis puts you into a trance-like state where you lose consciousness and awareness. This is a fear of many people, based on the premise of Myth 1: that hypnosis is mind control. Some people fear that by entering this state they will lose awareness of what is being said to them, become unconscious and unresponsive to their surroundings.

The Truth: Hypnosis is not a state of unconsciousness.

Hypnosis is often likened to being completely absorbed in a daydream, and although some clients will not consciously retain all that is discussed in a session, generally the key elements of the sessions will be recalled.

As we now know, hypnosis is a state of heightened awareness and focused attention. It is due to this heightened focus of attention that clients may well become less aware of their immediate surroundings, however brain studies show they are fully conscious, they also have an awareness of what is being said and have the ability to process thoughts and respond to their surroundings if so required. Clients can come out of hypnosis at any point and will certainly do so should they choose to or need to. Overall, the hypnotic experience is often described as being deeply comfortable and empowering.

Myth 3: Only a certain type of person can be hypnotised.

It is commonly believed that hypnosis only works on a select group of individuals who are either gullible or highly suggestible. This misconception along with the negative connotation it creates gives the false impression that hypnotherapy is only for the weak minded and therefore inaccessible to the majority of people. This misconception is also believed by some to be a fixed and unchangeable position.

The Truth: Hypnosis is one of the most natural states known to man and It has been practiced for thousands of years by many cultures. The main provisors are that the person is willing and open to the process. It is a voluntary state that almost everyone can enter to some degree if they choose to do so.

If you have ever become lost in a daydream or been immersed in a good book, then you have most certainly experienced a state of hypnotic trance to some degree. Likewise, if you have ever drifted off to sleep, or indeed woken up again, you have transitioned through the state of consciousness residing somewhere between wakefulness and sleep, known as the perfectly natural Hypnogogic state.

The effectiveness of any hypnotic session will be determined by many factors, not least of all rapport, trust and the skill of the practitioner who is trained to direct therapy specifically toward the needs of the client.

Myth 4: Hypnosis Is a form of Magic.

The idea that hypnosis is a "magical" solution that will fix all presenting problems is another common misconception.

Some individuals approach hypnotherapy with unrealistic expectations, believing that they are passive in the process, and the hypnotherapist has some magical power to solve all problems. This falls into the belief system that hypnosis is somehow applied or done to them and a single session is all it will take to instantly resolve any issue including long standing habits or emotional issues.

The Truth: Hypnosis is not magic.

Sound familiar?

Hypnotherapy is a therapeutic process that is done *with* the client, not *to* the client. It therefore requires the client to get involved and to actively participate in and be committed to the process.

Transformation can sometimes be rapid and profound; however, change is a process which is often most effective when combined with patience and persistence. New habit formation and lasting change requires conscious awareness, practice and appropriate follow-up sessions.

Myth 5: Hypnosis Is Dangerous

Some people have concerns about the nature of hypnosis, worrying that it might have harmful side effects, or worse still they may get stuck in trance. This fear is often generated by stories emanating from our friends in the movie industry or stage show performers who benefit from you believing these sensational popular narratives.

The Truth: Hypnosis is a safe and natural process. It is no more dangerous than meditation, deep breathing or daydreaming. Like meditation or daydreaming however, hypnosis must always only be entered into when you are in a safe environment to do so.

When it comes to your safety, It is also important to ensure your hypnotherapist is a well-trained ethical practitioner. Clients need to ensure they do their research and choose a reputable hypnotherapist who has undergone the required education and maintains accepted industry standards.

In Australia, The Australian Hypnotherapists' Association provides such standards and ensures all practitioners who are on the AHA Hypnotherapy Register meet the highest industry standards, abide by national codes of ethics and conduct and maintain annual Association requirements for effective therapists in this field.

With the right practitioner, hypnotherapy is safe and effective.

Myth 6: Hypnosis Can Make You Reveal Secrets

This is another common concern, also based in the unfounded belief that hypnosis is a state in which you have no control. This belief leads to a fear that the client will disclose hidden secrets, or worse, be induced to disclose personal or sensitive information. Naturally this can cause a great deal of anxiety and may deter clients from seeking hypnotherapeutic interventions.

The Truth: At all times the client is in complete control and will not disclose hidden secrets or the details of their internet banking whilst in a state of hypnosis, unless of course they have a desire to do so.

Again, I reiterate, hypnosis is a voluntary state in which you cannot be forced to reveal anything you do not wish to share. Foundational to the therapeutic relationship are trust and non-judgement. Clients are only encouraged to share that which is relevant to their healing journey.

Myth 7: Hypnosis Is a Form of Sleep

The word "hypnosis" was derived from the Greek word 'hypnos', meaning sleep, and for all intents and purposes a hypnotic state may resemble sleep to anyone looking on, however hypnosis is not sleep, and this misconception has further contributed to the myth that you are not in control during hypnosis.

The Truth: Clients may appear deeply relaxed during a hypnotherapy session; however, the reality is that their minds are highly active and their attention is focused. Contrary to sleep, a hypnotic state may often be described as a state of "hyper-awareness," in which the powerful subconscious part of the mind becomes more active and receptive to acceptable therapeutic suggestions.

Hypnotherapy involves active participation from the client who can respond to questioning, garner insights, recall memories and access resources to find solutions to presenting issues.

Myth 8: Hypnotherapy Is the Same as Stage Hypnosis

Certainly not!

While both forms of hypnosis involve an altered state of awareness and suggestion, the context and intention are vastly different.

The Truth: Stage hypnosis is for the purpose of entertainment only. Although it may often be confused with therapeutic hypnosis it is not created for therapeutic benefit. Its purpose may certainly be to promote the illusion of control on the part of the hypnotist, with theatrical statements like "Sleep now" indicating the willingness of the obedient participant to immediately submit to the will of the hypnotist. Although we now know that hypnosis is not sleep, the illusion of sleep and loss of control on the part of the volunteer, created in such situations furthers the audience's incorrect belief and therefore the intended deception is successfully created.

The context of stage hypnosis suggestions are often inclined to be dramatic providing maximum entertainment for the audience. Participants in stage hypnosis are typically pre-selected by the hypnotist for their displayed suggestibility and willingness to participate in the performance.

Therapeutic hypnosis on the other hand is an evidence based collaborative process that is goal directed to help individuals make positive changes in their thoughts, feelings and behaviours. It is facilitated by a therapeutic practitioner specifically trained in providing therapy during a hypnotic state. Therapy based on skilfully designed suggestions with a purpose to empower the client, are administered during the hypnotic state of heightened awareness, and at all times the client is conscious and in complete control.

Hypnotherapy is not magic, or manipulation, and should never be portrayed as such. It is about collaboration, awareness, and tapping into the power and potential of the human mind and body. It is always a deeply respectful, client-centred practice with a focus on healing and personal growth.

Myth 9: I will behave in embarrassing ways.

You will not behave in embarrassing ways unless of course you really wish to do so. As we have already ascertained, in hypnosis you are in complete control.

The Truth : This is a myth that serves a purpose for those who use hypnosis to earn their living from stage show or other types of performances. In all honesty many people enjoy participating in these performances, and many people enjoy watching the entertainment. Clearly both parties are getting some value from this incorrect assumption, however the reality as we now clearly understand, is that the hypnotist cannot make the participant do anything against their will.

Myth 10: Hypnosis Is only a Last Resort

Some people view hypnosis as a "last resort" therapy, to be tried only after other methods have failed. Indeed, I may say that many of my own clients who have experienced intractable issues for years and have exhausted all other avenues, have done exactly this, to finally experience relief after just a few short sessions of clinical hypnotherapy.

However, this 'last resort' perception undermines the reputation of hypnotherapy as a legitimate and potent first-line approach.

The Truth: clinical hypnotherapy is a versatile, evidence-based practice that can be used in combination with other therapies. It can also be utilised independently as a stand-alone treatment when practiced by well-trained clinical hypnotherapists. Research continues to show evidence that it is a particularly effective modality for many common mental health issues, such as anxiety, depression, stress management, insomnia, low self-esteem just to name a few. Its applications continue to grow. As clinical hypnotherapy has the ability to deal with subconscious underlying issues that may be driving the symptoms experienced, clients may certainly benefit from considering clinical hypnotherapy earlier rather than later.

The pervasive myths and misconceptions surrounding hypnotherapy have endured in the modern era for hundreds of years creating fear and scepticism. These myths have, and continue to, prevent clinical hypnotherapy from being seen as the legitimate and transformative therapeutic approach to healing and self-empowerment we know it to be.

With the passage of time these myths will dissipate. As more people experience this transformative therapy and share their successful experiences, the way will be paved for greater acceptance and understanding of this remarkable and enduring therapeutic approach.

Chapter Four

A BRIEF HISTORY OF HYPNOSIS: FROM ANCIENT RITUALS TO MODERN HEALING

Hypnosis has a history that is as rich and varied as humanity itself. From its roots in ancient civilisations' healing practices to its more recent integration in many mainstream medical practices, hypnotherapy is now viewed by many as an accepted and respected therapeutic field of study.

Understanding the history of hypnosis can help to illuminate the enduring power of the human mind to heal and transform.

Origins steeped in history indicate that the earliest recorded use of hypnosis, or practices resembling hypnosis date back thousands of years.

Astoundingly, one of the earliest references to hypnotic states can be found in the Ebers Papyrus, an ancient Egyptian medical text dating back to around 1550 BCE. This document describes the use of "temple sleep," a ritual in which individuals would enter sacred spaces to undergo healing processes facilitated by Priests. These Priests would guide the participants into trance-like states through rhythmic chanting and ritualistic ceremonial practices.

In ancient Greece and Rome hypnosis found its place within the temples of Asclepius, the god of healing. Individuals who were seeking relief from ailments would come to these temples to undergo a process in which they entered a dream-like state. Again, as in ancient Egypt, this was generally facilitated by prayer, chanting, and guided visualisation. The Greeks believed these states allowed divine intervention to heal the body and mind.

Hippocrates (approx. 460 BCE) known as the "Father of Modern Medicine," also grasped the underlying concepts related to the power of the mind in healing, long before modern science could verify it. Contrary to the popular doctrines of the time, he believed that illness was not a punishment from God, rather a result of natural causes. Despite not practicing hypnosis as we know it today, he recognised the healing potential of suggestion, relaxation, and altered states of consciousness. His approach promoted holistically treating the whole person, mind and body, rather than just the individual symptoms. Here it is possible to observe many parallels between Hippocrates's vision of healing and the practice of modern hypnosis, which also seeks to treat the person holistically and addresses mind and body as not separate, rather as intricately linked.

The Roman physician Galen (129–216 AD) also recognised the power of suggestion and psychological states in influencing physical health, although his work was not explicitly labelled as hypnosis.

Hypnotic states were also integral to ancient Indian practices, particularly in meditation and yoga. The concept of "trance" or "samadhi" described in yogic philosophy aligns closely with modern understandings of hypnosis as a deeply focused, altered state of consciousness.

During the Middle Ages, the use of hypnotic techniques shifted primarily into religious and spiritual practices. Monks, mystics, and shamans employed chanting, repetitive prayer, and meditation to induce trance-like states. These practices were believed to facilitate communication with the divine, leading to mystical experiences and spiritual or physical healing.

Unfortunately, due to the rise of religious doctrine at this time, practices that led to altered states of conscious awareness were viewed with great suspicion by the Church. Many of these practices were therefore outlawed and thus were practiced in secrecy. This fact led to them subsequently becoming associated with witchcraft or heresy which contributed to even more suppression in many parts of the world.

By the 18th century we can observe a turning point in the history of hypnosis. It now began to emerge as a more formalised practice. A shift could be observed where separation was occurring away from religious doctrine or mystical contexts.

Around this time a pivotal figure in the history of hypnosis, Franz Anton Mesmer, was born. Mesmer was an Austrian physician who believed in the concept of "animal magnetism." He believed that an invisible magnetic fluid existed within the body and that imbalances in this fluid caused illness. Mesmer was known to originally experiment with using iron magnets to treat illness. He subsequently used techniques such as magnetic passes or hand movements, and verbal suggestions to "realign" this energy, inducing trance-like states in his patients.

Mesmer's theory of animal magnetism was eventually discredited; however, Mesmer's work had a large influence on the future direction of hypnosis. His legacy continues to live on in the term that many of you have heard "mesmerism," which is viewed as a precursor to modern hypnosis.

Moving forward in time, Scottish surgeon James Braid (1795 – 1860) is thought to have first used the term "hypnosis." The origin of which came from the Greek word 'Hypnos,' meaning sleep. This was because Braid initially incorrectly believed hypnosis was a sleep-like state. He later clarified that hypnosis was not sleep, rather a state of focused attention and heightened suggestibility. Here, I'm sure you will notice, we can begin to see a very close connection to current definitions, and this brings us a little closer to our modern understanding of hypnosis.

Braid did his best to distance himself and his theory from the previous work of Franz Anton Mesmer. This was due to the widespread negative opinions of the medical and scientific community surrounding the practice of mesmerism at the time. By the time Braid began practicing hypnosis in the 1840s, mesmerism had largely been discredited. Braid's work therefore established hypnosis as a legitimate tool for therapeutic and medical purposes.

After this time, Scottish surgeon James Esdaile (1808-1859) utilised hypnosis to induce anaesthesia, this was naturally long before the advent of chemical anaesthesia. His work became a vital process for the management of pain and surgical procedures in the early 19th century. He is credited with performing over 300 major operations in India, including amputations. Patients are reported to have felt little to no pain. Despite this remarkable success, the use of hypnosis as an anaesthetic was quickly discontinued with the advent of ether in 1846.

Jean-Martin Charcot (1825–1893) also had an impact on the development and recognition of the practice of hypnosis. He was a French neurologist who studied hypnosis extensively in the treatment of hysteria which was originally considered a physical ailment. His work was controversial; however, it brought hypnosis to the attention of the medical community.

Sigmund Freud (1856–1939) also began using hypnosis in his practice to access repressed memories. He later shifted his focus to free association, however his early work demonstrated hypnosis's ability to reach the subconscious mind, which further influenced the development of modern psychotherapy.

Then in the early 20th century the great Milton H. Erickson (1901–1980) revolutionised the field of hypnosis. His innovative techniques emphasised the use of indirect suggestion, storytelling, metaphor and rapport to guide clients into trance states. Erickson's approach, known as Ericksonian hypnosis, remains a cornerstone of modern hypnotherapy, utilising client individuality, creativity and resources to achieve their therapeutic goals.

Today, hypnosis is recognised as a powerful tool for psychological and physical healing. Research continues to demonstrate its efficacy in treating conditions such as chronic pain, anxiety, depression, and trauma, to name but a few applications.

Organisations such as the **Australian Hypnotherapists' Association,** one of the oldest hypnotherapy associations in the world, and certainly the oldest in Australia, continue to lead the way in raising awareness and clinical standards for the ethical practice of clinical hypnotherapy not only in Australia, but around the world.

As a clinical hypnotherapist heavily involved in the professional transformation of clinical hypnotherapy in Australia, I often reflect on the ancient rituals and practices that paved the way for modern hypnotherapy, emphasising the universal and enduring nature of this modality.

As we continue to seek recognition based on the rising body of evidential research, it is important to remember where we have come from, so we can look forward with anticipation and hope for the future. As Sir Isaac Newton once said, "If I have seen further, it is by standing upon the shoulders of giants".

As practitioners and clients, we stand on the shoulders of the mystics, healers, and pioneers who recognised the power of the mind and dared to explore its depths. By honouring this history, we deepen our connection to the practice and embrace its possibilities for the future. Therefore, let us all continue to stand on the shoulders of the giants that came before us, in our desire to further advance this powerfully transformative therapy.

This is not an exhaustive list of all of those who have been influential in the development of the practice of hypnotherapy as we know it today, however it gives us a broad understanding. The evolving history of hypnosis is an ongoing testament to humanity's enduring quest for self-understanding and healing.

From the sacred temples of ancient civilisations to the clinical settings of today, hypnosis has continued to evolve while retaining its core purpose: to harness the mind's incredible power and potential to heal and transform.

I believe hypnosis to be the metaphoric bridge that connects us to the wisdom of the past, traversing the scientific underpinnings of the present and leading the way forward toward the creative potential of the future, offering us all a pathway to healing that transcends time.

Chapter Five

THE SILENT BURDEN - UNDERSTANDING STRESS AND THE TRANSFORMATIVE POWER OF HYPNOTHERAPY

Now that we have delved into the past, let us bring our focus into the present.

You might wonder why I've chosen to begin this section of the book with a focus on stress when exploring the mechanisms and applications of hypnotherapy. The reason is straightforward: chronic stress is a defining feature of modern life and a common thread underlying many of the challenges individuals face today, both personally and collectively. As you continue through this book, you may notice a common theme. Stress is that theme, and it is often a contributing factor in the 'A' to 'Z' of issues that bring people to hypnotherapy, ranging from agoraphobia to feeling zapped of energy and everything in between. Throughout this book, we will examine how stress plays a significant role in ill health and how hypnotherapy can offer meaningful relief, restoration and often resolution.

What can you do?

The key may lie in enhancing your ability to focus more mindfully on your daily experiences, what you're doing, thinking, and feeling.

Simple, isn't it? Yet, it is often so challenging. By becoming observers of our own experiences, we can start to see and understand that regardless of the issue at hand, very similar principles are at play when seeking a solution. This insight proves invaluable for us as therapists.

When we recognise that the impacts of stress will manifest in our client's bodies in numerous damaging ways, we will need to set about alleviating this causative factor. We can achieve this through many processes that have their roots in physiology, psychology and neurology. We will further explore this theme throughout the pages of this book, and as we do we can begin to create a framework for fostering holistic health and harmony within ourselves, and our clients. I discuss this principle in my book the *Health and Happiness Handbook* along with its companion journal which provides many examples of practical ways to alleviate stress and create desirable outcomes.

As you will hear me say many times throughout this book, in order to treat an issue, we need to really understand it. So, what is Stress? This word we hear constantly is an experience that some of us know too well. It can creep into our minds without conscious awareness, and our ever-responsive bodies will oblige by obediently and immediately changing our physiology and the circulating chemistry in our bodies, all with an intention to keep us safe from the unknown and in many cases unreal danger.

This resulting shift in our chemistry and our physiology, impacts how we think, feel and perceive the world around us. When this response is warranted and appropriate, it can save our lives, however when it is allowed free reign to run amuck, like a badly behaved puppy bounding from disaster to disaster, undermining our every thought feeling and emotion, it can feel like trouble awaits us around every corner.

In the latter example, the unhealthy imagined scenarios are embodied by us and produce an often damaging 'Allostatic load" which creates wear and tear affecting every organ and system including the brain. This habitual 'stress response' often leads to predictable chronic and cumulative body system damage. When left unchecked debilitating anxiety, can result, sometimes resulting in Generalised Anxiety Disorder (GAD). When this happens, the unrelenting stress response may continue to dictate our every move.

The good news is that with the benefit of hypnotherapy it is possible to reprogram the mind and body to respond differently to the normal stressors, and more importantly to the imagined stressors, of life effectively. When this happens you create the space and environment that allows your body and / or that of your clients to heal, restore and repair rather than continuing the path of deteriorating physical and emotional health, which probably brought them to see you in the first place.

An important truth to remember:

It is not what happens to us that creates our stress, it is what we *think* about what happens to us that creates stress.

This is not a new concept.

Mark Twain is well known for saying; " I have had a lot of worries in my life, most of which never happened."

Long before this Michel de Montaigne, French Philosopher; born 1533, was known to have said "My life has been full of terrible misfortunes, most of which never happened."

Another well-known historic figure Lucius Annaeus Seneca; Roman philosopher and one of the most influential thinkers of ancient Rome said, "We suffer more often in imagination than in reality."

These are all powerful reminders that much of our distress is created by our own very vivid and equally powerful imagination. It also becomes apparent that this has been known for a millennium, and although these and many other famous quotes abound, many are yet to learn how to master their thoughts to gain emotional and physical peace and clarity.

What we now know with the benefit of modern science and technology, which these insightful forward thinkers of the past may not have known, is that prolonged and unchecked stress is damaging to every system in your body. The effects of which manifest differently in different people, creating a variety of presenting issues that may be physical, emotional or chemical, and will quietly undermine the health and well-being of the recipient.

Let us now explore how hypnotherapy can offer a profound solution, to not only manage stress, but to transform the way we think, feel and experience life itself.

When we allow our fertile imagination to travel directly to the worst scenario, that thing that you dread may happen, even though it is *not* happening, we activate our Sympathetic Nervous System. This is often referred to as 'Fight-Flight-Freeze Mode' or 'Stress Mode' and is characterised by a sudden and immediate release of chemicals and by the activation of physiological processes all designed to save our lives. During this state the body is immediately prepared to either run away from the impending danger, fight to defend itself or become very still in the hope of going unnoticed.

For the purpose of this book, I will call this 'Fight-Flight Mode'.

When we explore the fight-flight mode, we notice that human beings are unique in our ability to mentally manufacture stress and sustain it without any actual physical threat present. In fact, we are the only species in the world who can very effectively turn this powerful chemical and physical response on in a millisecond, with our thoughts alone, in the complete absence of any real danger. Think about that for a moment. Some people can live in "stress" mode for a majority of the time, creating a state that many know all too well as Anxiety.

We all have the ability to trigger fight-flight mode when we worry about things that are not happening; things that may never happen. The 'what if' concerns, the looming deadlines at work, pending exams, phone messages, and emails we have yet to attend to, and the list goes on.

According to Beyond Blue approximately 3.3 million Australians are living with Anxiety. This aligns with the Australian Bureau of statistics National Study of Health and Wellbeing (2020-2022) which reports 17.2% of Australians aged between 16-85 have experienced anxiety disorder in the previous 12 months. I would postulate that quite probably there are many more who remain unreported and undiagnosed.

When an anxious state becomes our new 'normal' there are predictable physical and chemical outcomes that occur in the body and brain to accommodate the circulating stress chemistry surging through our bodies and the accompanying stressful feelings. When we consider that the powerful subconscious mind cannot tell the difference between reality or imagination, it is not surprising that it responds as though our distressing musings are true. The result is over time we see the brain's stress centre, the amygdala, becoming enlarged, while simultaneously other areas of the brain shrink. During periods of prolonged stress, the hippocampus – the area of the brain that stores memories, and the prefrontal cortex area that deals with decision making, working memory and impulse control are both reduced in size.

If that hasn't caught your attention, I will also tell you that stress kills existing brain cells and slows regeneration of new brain cells. These changes effectively wire the brain for more stress and consequently a new base line is created. Now we are wired for stress.

Most people presenting to the hypnotherapy clinic for this reason will have already taken ownership of this state by saying *"I'm stressed-out"*, *"I am an anxious person"* or *"I'm always stressed"*. Here we can see the self-fulfilling prophecy playing out to be true. The more we feel stressed, the more stressed thoughts we have, and the more stressed thoughts we have the more we feel stressed, and so the stress loop continues.

This is probably a good time to reflect on the basic principles of neuroplasticity, and for any of you who have studied neuroscience in any capacity you may recall 'Hebb's Rule' ***Neurons that fire together, wire together***. The longer you choose to linger in the stress state which triggers activation of your "fight-flight-mode", the more you wire your brain for that state.

You may ask, why is it that we have this dominant, very powerful and often damaging response? The answer is simple. When our ancestors were faced with real danger, a wild animal or a sudden attack, their survival depended on the very rapid activation of the fight-or-flight response. The brain would quickly detect the threat and release a surge of adrenaline and cortisol, increasing heart rate, sharpening focus, and preparing the body for immediate action. But once the danger had passed, the system naturally returned to balance, giving the body time to rest, recover, and reset.

To be clear, the fight-or-flight response is not inherently negative. In fact, in more modern times, this response continues to be an essential and life-saving reaction that you absolutely want to activate automatically in the presence of real danger, such as when touching a hot surface or stepping into the path of a speeding car. In such moments, this rapid physiological shift is critical to your survival and may just save your life.

In the case of our ancestors, right through to modern times, this response was only ever intended to be short-term and situation specific. It was never meant to be a constant state of being. Why? Living in a prolonged state of fight-or-flight can and does lead to significant harm and is responsible for so many of the conditions that will present to the hypnotherapy clinic, which is why we are exploring it in this book.

This is where the concept of allostatic load becomes relevant. Allostatic load refers to the cumulative wear and tear on the body caused by chronic stress and repeated activation of the stress response. Elevated allostatic load has been linked to a disturbing range of health issues that can be physical, emotional and / or behavioral, including:

- A surge in stress chemicals in the body
- Increased / shallow breathing
- Increased heart rate
- Thick sticky blood / ready to clot if you are injured
- High blood lipids / fats / glucose levels
- Hypertension (high blood pressure)
- Increased hardening of the arteries
- Cardiovascular disease
- Damage to the peripheral vascular system (veins and arteries)
- Increased risk of Stroke and Heart attack
- Greater risk of developing diabetes
- General body pain and discomfort
- Increase in muscle pains
- Fibromyalgia
- Weight gain
- Reduced bone density
- Increased frailty
- Digestive issues such as: Nausea, constipation, indigestion, irritable bowel.
- Prolonged brain exposure to Neurotoxic Stress chemicals
- Thinning of brain's grey matter
- Impaired cognitive function and cognitive decline
- Damaged brain cells over time
- Reduced neurogenesis (creation of new brain cells)
- Increase in size and function of the brain's stress centre
- Brain rewires itself for more stress.
- Memory loss
- Increased predisposition to dementia
- Increased inflammation
- Reduced function of the immune system
- Reduced function of the reproductive system
- Rapid ageing of our DNA associated with 'telomere' shortening
- Visible Ageing – reduced peripheral circulation
- Higher rates of psychological disorders

- Increased anxiety and depression
- Elevated self-reported stress
- Increased alcohol abuse
- Increased drug abuse
- Irritability
- Anger outbursts
- Increased domestic violence
- Increased anti-social behaviours
- Isolation
- Restlessness
- Feelings of overwhelm
- Increased relationship issues
- Insomnia
- Rumination

Many people are often surprised by just how extensive the impact of chronic stress and elevated allostatic load can be across all aspects of physical, behavioural, and psychological health. This list is by no means exhaustive. The evidence is compelling and by now, you may agree that taking steps to reduce your allostatic load is not only wise, but essential for long-term health and well-being.

This is precisely where hypnotherapy becomes a valuable clinical tool. By guiding an individual into a deep state of focused attention, hypnotherapy can be utilised to activate the parasympathetic branch of the autonomic nervous system, the system responsible for 'rest and digest' functions. This deliberate physiological shift counters the sympathetic nervous system's 'fight-or-flight' response and promotes a decrease in heart rate, blood pressure, respiratory rate, and the secretion of stress hormones such as cortisol and adrenaline.

Over time and with needed repetition and regular engagement, hypnotherapy can support the recalibration of the nervous system, making it less reactive to perceived threats and more resilient to daily stressors. By combining activation of the parasympathetic nervous system with goal-oriented subconscious suggestions, hypnotherapy offers a dual approach that can alleviate the immediate effects of stress whilst simultaneously addressing its underlying causes. The outcome is a reduced allostatic load and improved long-term mental, emotional, and physical health.

THE MINDS ROLE IN STRESS

Although the body experiences stress physically and chemically, its roots lie in the mind. The way we perceive a situation determines whether it triggers stress or not. For example, two people can experience the very same challenge such as public speaking, yet one may feel exhilarated, energised, and confident, while the other may be crippled by anxiety long before the event has even occurred.

Now that we understand the body can enter a state of stress almost instantly triggered by thoughts alone, even in the absence of any real threat, it becomes increasingly plausible to consider that we may also have the capacity to shift out of stress mode using the power of the mind in a similarly immediate and intentional way.

The good news is that not only is it possible to deactivate the stress response and reduce the allostatic load your body has been carrying, but it is also entirely achievable to rewire the brain, promoting greater calm, emotional regulation, and a more positive outlook over time.

The body is complex, that is true. It is a remarkable combination of systems and finely tuned responses designed to keep us safe. Therefore, when we learn to speak to the body in language that the body understands, we can hijack these natural responses and use them to instantly create calm and clarity. When the stress response is no longer dominating, it becomes far easier to move toward the outcomes we desire.

This is where hypnotherapy truly offers a unique and powerful difference. While many forms of stress management focus on external strategies, like exercise, relaxation techniques, or lifestyle adjustments, hypnotherapy goes deeper. It works directly with the subconscious mind, where long-held stress responses and belief patterns are stored. And this comes with a powerful bonus, and that is, as we now know, the subconscious doesn't distinguish between real and imagined experiences. What this means is the body can and will respond just as strongly to a vivid mental image as it does to an actual event. We observe this principle in the previously mentioned case of public speaking. The images held by you can heighten your anxiety long before you've even stepped on stage. However, this same imaginative potential, when harnessed in the right way, can be used to create calm, build confidence, and guide you toward your best possible outcome.

One of the most important concepts I ask every one of my clients to embrace is based on the following principle:

The moment you become aware of anything, you are immediately in a position of choice, what you choose in that moment will determine your outcomes.

HYPNOTHERAPY AND REWIRING THE STRESS RESPONSE

Hypnotherapy is a safe, deeply therapeutic practice that harnesses the natural power of the mind to create lasting change.

The subconscious mind is where our habits, beliefs, and emotional responses are stored. It is also where stress patterns can take firm root. Through hypnosis, we can access this part of the mind, which is often not visible to the conscious mind, and rewrite the programs that have previously dictated our responses.

So how does hypnotherapy help?

As many stress responses have been learned over time, hypnotherapy can help in shifting our perspective.

For example, If we grow up in an environment where any kind of stress response is the norm, the body learns to remain in a heightened state of alertness. One could argue that this itself is a state of trance and perhaps explains why some of these patterns and habits become so firmly entrenched. Thus, the person experiencing the stress begins to live with an elevated stress baseline, whereby they may never fully relax. We would say that they have become neurologically wired for stress.

Hypnotherapy, through its ability to bypass the critical conscious mind helps to gently reprogram the subconscious mind, allowing the same person to take a different perspective from a calm vantage point and interpret situations with more clarity. Instead of triggering the same old stress response, the brain learns a new, more effective response.

Hypnosis and relaxation are both very effective in triggering activation of the parasympathetic nervous system, sometimes referred to as the Relaxation Response, which is the direct opposite to the stress state. Now although we have ascertained that hypnosis is not relaxation in and of itself, relaxation can certainly play a crucial role in helping a stressed individual effectively reach a hypnotic state, and many practitioners use relaxation techniques to do just that.

As we have stated, the mind can create stress. That said, the mind can also induce profound relaxation when given a different set of instructions. When a person is guided into a deeply relaxed state utilising progressive muscle relaxation and breath work, activation of the parasympathetic nervous system occurs, and hypnosis often easily follows.

Hypnotherapy can be utilised to guide individuals into even deeper states of hypnosis using carefully constructed language allowing the body to further release tension, lower cortisol levels and other stress chemistry leading to a restoration of homeostatic equilibrium; balance is returned. When practiced, it is a process that begins to retrain the nervous system, making calmness more accessible in everyday life.

Once a person reaches a state of hypnosis, they can begin to investigate the underlying root causes of their stress response. Stress often stems from past wounds, unresolved grief, repressed memories, or entrenched beliefs about self-worth. Hypnotherapy offers a safe environment to gently guide an individual below the surface to uncover what triggers their stress. By identifying the true source of our stress and approaching it with care and compassion, significant changes can occur. This process enables healing at a deeper level, ultimately allowing true transformation to take place.

When stress is addressed, improved sleep often follows. Insomnia will have its own chapter in this book because one of the most common side effects of elevated stress is disrupted sleep. Stress can lead to the mind racing, and the body remains in daytime mode. Daytime mode is characterised by your brain humming with beta brain waves, fast, focused, and sharp. In this state restorative sleep becomes elusive. Hypnotherapy can help quiet the mental chatter, guiding individuals to experience deeper, more restful sleep. A positive cycle of healing can be achieved during restful sleep, and as stress levels reduce naturally, a space for the body to repair itself is created.

Reducing stress also has positive effects on the functioning of the brain, and again hypnosis facilitates this shift. When you enter a hypnotic state, your brain shifts into a more relaxed frequency, most commonly theta waves. This will be discussed further in the next chapter: The Brain in Trance: The Neuroscience of hypnotherapy.

One of the most empowering elements of the hypnotherapeutic process for stress reduction is the opportunity for individuals to feel empowered and regain control over their lives. Self-hypnosis is often integrated into client therapy sessions between scheduled appointments. This aspect is crucial, as it enables individuals to feel they have the ability to affect their own changes and enhance their outcomes. By actively participating in the process and practicing effective tools, clients can navigate life with greater ease and resilience.

A CASE STUDY: SAM'S STORY

Sam, a 42-year-old teacher, came to hypnotherapy feeling exhausted and overwhelmed. She had been experiencing chronic stress for years balancing work, family, and personal expectations, all of which had left her feeling depleted. Her body showed the not unexpected effects: frequent headaches, digestive discomfort, and insomnia.

Through hypnotherapy, Sam began to uncover deep-seated patterns of perfectionism and self-criticism. Her stress wasn't just about external pressure it was rooted in a belief that she was never doing enough.

By working with her subconscious mind, she was able to explore and reframe this belief and replace it with a more supportive mindset. Ongoing sessions helped her retrain her stress response, activating calmness instead of panic, and creating a solution-focused state of attention. Over time, her headaches faded, her sleep and digestion improved, and perhaps most importantly, she began to feel joy again.

It's essential to recognise that the improvements Sam experienced did not occur after a single hypnotherapy session. Change came through her awareness of old patterns and habits, as well as her commitment to putting into practice her new mindset whenever she found herself reverting to old thoughts, feelings, and behaviours. Awareness is crucial for change, and consistent practice is necessary. Self-hypnosis and a solution-focused approach are valuable tools that can be used daily as needed.

Sam integrated the following principles into her daily routines.

Progressive Relaxation: Systematically relaxing each muscle group helps release stored tension and signals to the body that you are safe, and it is safe to relax.

Daily self-hypnosis: Spending just five to ten minutes a day in a relaxed state with a positive, solution-focused attention—reinforcing new neural pathways.

Breath Awareness: Using deep, controlled breathing which activated her parasympathetic nervous system, paying particular attention to the long slow exhalation which can instantly calm the body and reduce stress in real-time.

Mindful Reframing: When stressful thoughts surfaced, Sam took a moment to pause, notice, challenge, and reframe the situation. This effectively alters the body's response. By asking herself if this was a helpful thought / feeling or behaviour that would take her to her desired outcome, Sam was able to interrupt and prevent the previous automatic stress reaction.

By becoming more aware of how stress affects the body and the mind, we can utilise hypnotherapy to rewire our previously hard-wired responses. Stress may be an inevitable part of life, but suffering under its weight is optional.

Awareness is the key to creating the changes we seek. With awareness we can move from a place of previous automatic stress-based reactions to a more considered response set; one of balance, clarity, and calm. From this calmer vantage point, we can utilise self-hypnotic practices every day to activate a more goal-oriented mindset, which the subconscious mind will respond to.

We know that by stepping into a more solution focused state and imagining it as if it has already been achieved, we are literally rewiring the brain for a different response. The more we engage in this practice, the stronger our response will become, eventually making it our default reaction, and this was exactly what Sam noticed. She felt empowered by the understanding that she could now shape her outcomes through awareness, insight and importantly a non-judgmental attitude towards her old habits. Most importantly, she embraced repetition. By continually applying these practices, her results became a brilliant illustration of what is possible when her powerful mind and body function in harmony.

Through the power of the mind, we have the ability not just to manage stress, but to transform the way we experience life itself. And this is where true healing begins.

Chapter Six

THE BRAIN IN TRANCE: THE NEUROSCIENCE OF HYPNOTHERAPY

In the quiet space of a hypnotherapy session, something quite extraordinary is happening beneath the surface. While the client may appear still, their mind is alive with activity, as neural circuits reconfigure themselves in response to suggestion, imagery, and metaphor. The science of hypnotherapy is a story of connection, between mind and body, conscious and subconscious, therapist and client. And at the heart of this connection is the brain.

In recent years, advancements in neuroscience have provided remarkable insights into the workings of hypnotherapy, revealing that this ancient practice is fundamentally rooted in biology. Hypnotherapy is not a trick or a mystical experience; rather, it is a neurobiological process with measurable effects on the brain. To comprehend its transformative potential, we must explore what occurs in the brain during trance, how hypnotherapy leverages neuroplasticity, and why it is uniquely positioned to facilitate healing and change.

Before delving into this however, let us debunk a prevailing misconception that persists despite compelling evidence to the contrary. The enduring metaphor of the "lizard brain," based on Paul MacLean's triune brain theory, inaccurately posits that the brain evolved in three distinct layers: reptilian, limbic, and neocortical, each governing survival, emotion, and reasoning. Despite its continued usage in therapeutic and popular psychology, this model has been widely discredited. Contemporary neuroscience illustrates that the brain functions as an interconnected, dynamic system rather than a rigid evolutionary hierarchy (Luiz Pessoa, 2013).

Neuroplasticity, the brain's ability to reorganise itself in response to experiences, further challenges the notion of fixed, primitive brain regions. It underscores our inherent capacity to reshape emotional patterns, behaviours, and beliefs over time (Doidge, 2007). This understanding positions the brain as an adaptable system, uniquely designed for healing and growth. Current research also emphasises that complex behaviours arise from dynamic interactions throughout the brain, not isolated parts. Thus, the triune brain serves more as a metaphor than an accurate representation of brain structure and evolution. Now that we have a more accurate understanding of the brain and its functions, let us continue.

Hypnosis often described as a state of focused attention and heightened suggestibility, is so much more than a mental state. It is a neurological phenomenon. When a client enters trance, specific regions of the brain show distinct patterns of activity, as revealed by functional MRI (fMRI) and electroencephalogram (EEG) studies.

One of the most notable changes occurs in the default mode network (DMN). This network, which includes areas like the medial prefrontal cortex and posterior cingulate cortex, is responsible for self-referential thinking, that's our inner chatter, self-criticism, and ruminations. In hypnosis, activity in the DMN reduces, creating a quieter internal environment. In other words, the part of the brain that deals with judgement, quietens.

It has often been said over many years, prior to our ability to see into the functioning brain with the aid of technology, that hypnosis bypasses the 'critical faculty'. This, it appears, is precisely what happens in the brain in trance. This reduction allows clients to step outside of their habitual thought patterns and experience a sense of detachment from their usual, sometimes judgemental, narrative. When the DMN quietens down it can often also lead to a reduced sense of time, place and self, which as you may be aware, are characteristic of trance states.

At the same time, the anterior cingulate cortex (ACC), a region that plays a critical role in attention and decision-making, shows increased activity. This surge in activation corresponds to the deep concentration often reported by clients during hypnosis. It's as if the brain sharpens its focus, minimising distractions and aligning more closely with the therapeutic goals and directions.

Another pivotal region involved in the hypnotic state is the insula, which is tied to body awareness and emotions. During hypnosis, activity in the insula increases, strengthening the link between the mind and body. This heightened connection enables the experiential nature of hypnosis to expand and blossom. This helps explain why hypnotherapy is particularly effective for treating conditions such as chronic pain, as it enables clients to become more aware of, and more focused on, other physical sensations which can change how they perceive their discomfort.

When we bring all of this together, we start to understand the deeper shift that occurs during a hypnotic trance. The combined effects of these three distinct regions reveal that in hypnosis, there's a softening of self-judgment. At the same time, we unlock a clearer, more focused capacity for decision-making and can experience a profound, enriched connection between mind and body.

Hypnosis not only influences specific brain regions, it also induces changes in brainwave patterns. This happens as the conscious brain moves toward a deeper hypnotic state. The human brain operates on electrical rhythms categorised into five main types of brainwaves:

- Delta (0.5–4 Hz): Associated with deep sleep.

- Theta (4–8 Hz): Linked to deep relaxation, creativity, and access to the subconscious.
- Alpha (8–12 Hz): Representing a calm, meditative state.
- Beta (12–30 Hz): Associated with active thinking and alertness.
- Gamma (30–100 Hz): Tied to high-level cognitive functioning and insight.

During hypnosis, the brain predominantly enters a theta state, characterised by a slowing of brainwaves. This state allows for a heightened ability to access the deeper subconscious mind and is often considered optimal for hypnotherapy, as it can facilitate the safe exploration of memories, emotions, and beliefs that are typically stored beneath the level of conscious awareness.

The theta state is also linked to increased neuroplasticity, which is the brain's capacity to reorganise itself by forming new neural connections. This enhanced plasticity is noteworthy as it can help to explain why hypnotherapy can be very powerful in producing lasting changes. In short, what this means is, theta brainwaves provide a state that prepares the brain for change.

One of the most profound aspects of hypnotherapy is its ability to engage the subconscious mind. The subconscious mind, previously shrouded in mysticism and misunderstandings is now recognised to be the domain of the limbic system, the emotional centre of the brain. The limbic system includes structures like the amygdala, hippocampus, and hypothalamus, which govern emotions, memory, and the body's stress responses.

When we experience trauma, the amygdala becomes hyperactive, locking us into a state of hypervigilance. The hippocampus, responsible for processing and understanding memories, may fail to encode a traumatic event properly, leading to flashbacks or intrusive thoughts.

The mind and body encode this event as a potential threat and store the memory where it can be easily accessed, thus these trauma memories do not fade away as other memories can. We may call this a post traumatic event.

Hypnotherapy helps process such memories by soothing the amygdala while actively engaging the hippocampus in a safe and controlled manner. In this relaxed mental state, the therapist can use guided imagery, metaphors, and solution-focused suggestions to assist the client in processing these memories. This method fosters a supportive and, importantly, safe environment, allowing the client to reprocess and reframe disturbing memories. This helps them develop more suitable and acceptable responses, moving away from their previous emotional reactions.

For instance, a client with a fear of public speaking might revisit the origin of their fear in trance, seeing it not as an unchangeable truth but as a moment in time that can be rewritten. This reprocessing is supported by the prefrontal cortex, which remains active during hypnosis, allowing for critical thinking and emotional regulation.

Further to our discussion on stress in the previous chapter, the body's stress response is primarily regulated by the hypothalamic-pituitary-adrenal (HPA) axis, a key neuroendocrine system that governs the release of stress hormones such as cortisol. This response is vital for immediate survival, helping the body manage acute stress. However, prolonged or repeated activation of the HPA axis, as seen in chronic stress, can contribute to a range of health issues, including anxiety, depression, impaired immune function, and chronic pain.

Research indicates that hypnosis can influence the activity of the HPA axis. This often results in a reduction of cortisol levels and a shift toward activation of the parasympathetic nervous system; the state associated with rest and recovery. This physiological change not only fosters a sense of calm but also supports longer-term benefits such as enhanced emotional regulation, improved immune resilience, and reduced inflammation.

In fact, studies have found that hypnotherapy can alter the brain's pain pathways, reducing the perception of pain without relying on medication. It works by gently shifting the brain's response in areas that control both the physical sensation and the emotional impact of pain. By targeting both the emotional and physical components of pain, hypnotherapy offers relief that is both holistic and lasting. We will discuss this further in the chapter titled: Hypnotherapy for Pain Management.

At the heart of hypnotherapy's effectiveness lies the principle of neuroplasticity, the brain's natural capacity to reorganise, form new connections, and evolve throughout life. This flexibility is what allows us to break old habits, overcome challenges, and reshape the beliefs that may previously have held us back.

When someone is in a hypnotic state, the brain becomes more open to change due to the physiological shifts that we have discussed. The effects of these physiological changes in the brain can create an environment where a softening of the usual filters and resistances occur. This often allows for new, more supportive ways of thinking to take root. This is especially helpful for clients who have previously felt caught in cycles of self-doubt, fear, or unhelpful behaviours.

Take, for instance, a client who has spent many years believing, "I'm not good enough," a belief that has been reinforced through repetition and much focus of attention, which creates something akin to a deep groove in the brain's wiring. At this point we may remember Hebb's rule – "Neurons that fire together wire together" and this further reinforces the habitual thinking and feeling that has been keeping that belief firmly wired in place.

In hypnotherapy, new ideas, such as "I am capable" or "I belong" are introduced gently and vividly, inviting the client to imagine living from those truths. As these new thoughts are practised, the brain begins to strengthen these healthier pathways, while the old ones begin to weaken in a process known as synaptic pruning. The outcome isn't just a shift in mindset; it's a genuine transformation in how the brain responds, thinks, and feels.

Many other forms of therapy focus on the conscious mind. Hypnotherapy offers a unique approach. It goes beyond surface-level awareness to gently access the deeper, often overlooked realm of the subconscious. Traditional talk therapies generally engage the conscious mind, the part of our minds responsible for logic, reasoning, and reflection. In contrast, hypnotherapy guides clients into a deeper state where it is possible to explore the long-standing patterns, emotional memories, and automatic responses that are held there.

You might wonder why this makes such a profound difference. I would say that it's because, by conservative estimates, around 93% of our behaviours are driven by the subconscious. These are the automatic habits and patterns we follow daily, often without realising, often despite consciously wanting to change them. Hypnotherapy works at this subconscious level where these deeply rooted responses are stored, making meaningful change more accessible.

The blending of conscious insight with the subconscious potential to create change, often generates a powerful momentum that supports transformation. Instead of simply consciously understanding what needs to shift, clients begin to feel and observe change taking place in their body and mind. This creates a sense of integration that can be both immediate and lasting.

As neuroscience continues to advance, so too does our appreciation for what hypnotherapy can truly offer. With the help of modern tools like brain imaging, we're beginning to uncover how the hypnotic state affects specific neural circuits. At the same time, clinical research continues to explore its benefits across a range of conditions, from trauma and anxiety to chronic pain, addiction, digestive disorders and so much more.

However, what stands out most to any experienced hypnotherapist, is not just the science, but rather the human experience at the heart of it. Hypnotherapy is revealing itself to be a powerful tool which can be used to access the brain's natural ability to adapt and heal. In skilled hands, it becomes a meeting point where science, knowledge and deep intuitive wisdom intersect. A place where the client's attention is deliberately directed toward their intention, where the deep wisdom of the subconscious mind can be not only accessed, but fully embraced to create optimal and previously illusive outcomes.

As practitioners, we're not simply facilitating therapy in a hypnotic state, we're bearing witness to the brain's quiet, yet often extraordinary, capacity to reshape itself. This is real change from the inside – out. In that process, genuine change doesn't just feel possible, it is possible.

IN SUMMARY - HOW HYPNOTHERAPY INFLUENCES BRAIN FUNCTION

As mentioned above, recent advancements in neuroscience have illuminated how hypnotherapy affects brain function, offering a compelling scientific foundation for its therapeutic benefits. The following points are a summary and highlight many key findings:

Reduction in Default Mode Network (DMN) Activity

Hypnosis has been linked to decreased activity in the DMN, a brain network associated with self-referential thinking and mind-wandering. This reduction may enhance present-moment awareness and focused attention during therapy.

Enhanced Activation of the Anterior Cingulate Cortex (ACC)

Research shows increased activity in the ACC during hypnosis, a region involved in regulating attention and cognitive control. This aligns with the heightened focus and openness to suggestion commonly observed in hypnotic states.

Increased Engagement of the Insula

The insula, responsible for emotional awareness and interoception (the perception of internal bodily states), becomes more active during hypnosis. This may support the emotional insight and mind-body integration often experienced in hypnotherapy.

Elevation of Theta Brainwave Activity

Hypnosis is associated with an increase in theta wave activity (4–7 Hz), which corresponds with deep relaxation and enhanced access to the subconscious. This brainwave state supports receptivity for therapeutic suggestion.

Promotion of Neuroplasticity

Hypnotherapy may enhance neuroplasticity. This is the brain's capacity to form and reorganise neural pathways, allowing for lasting behavioural and cognitive shifts.

Engagement of the Limbic System

Increased activation of the limbic system, particularly the amygdala and hippocampus (key regions for emotion and memory), has been observed during hypnosis. This may facilitate emotional processing and trauma resolution.

Regulation of the Hypothalamic-Pituitary-Adrenal (HPA) Axis

Hypnosis appears to influence the HPA axis, reducing cortisol levels and calming the body's stress response. This supports its effectiveness in treating anxiety and stress-related conditions.

Altered Pain Perception

Functional neuroimaging has shown that hypnosis can change pain perception by modulating activity in areas such as the anterior cingulate cortex, thalamus, and somatosensory cortex. This helps explain its role in pain management.

Access to Conscious and Subconscious Processes

Hypnosis allows therapeutic access to both conscious awareness and subconscious processes, enabling interventions that work with ingrained beliefs, habits, and emotional responses.

Ongoing Advances in Hypnosis Research

Continued research using fMRI and EEG is expanding our understanding of the neural mechanisms involved in hypnosis, contributing to its broader clinical application.

~

From its faith-based beginnings, hypnotherapy has transitioned into a discipline backed by scientific evidence and technological advances. This evolution propels hypnotherapy into a new frontier, no longer relegated to the fringes or dismissed as pseudoscience. Today, robust research and cutting-edge technologies provide irrefutable evidence of its efficacy, demonstrating that hypnotherapy is a valid and powerful tool for lasting change grounded in neuroscience, physiology, and psychology. We are firmly established, and our results speak volumes.

Welcome to the new era of clinical hypnotherapy.

Chapter Seven

THE NEW STORY OF GENETICS: BIOPLASTICITY AND EPIGENETICS IN ACTION

When people think of genetics, they often picture a rigid, unchangeable code passed down through generations; a script set in stone that determines who we are. Yet, science now illuminates a more hopeful narrative. Surprising scientific discoveries in the fields of neuroplasticity, bioplasticity, and epigenetics now show that we are far more adaptable than once was believed.

As a Nurse and Midwife, I spent many years working in the area of Artificial Reproductive Technology (ART). Here, I studied genetic counselling, due to the nature of my work coordinating the genetic embryo biopsy program. The aim of which was to identify genetically abnormal embryos prior to implantation. Therefore, the area of genetics has always fascinated me. Now as a clinical hypnotherapist, I continue to be excited by the new scientific discoveries of epigenetics. I have often pondered: How much of our outcomes are predetermined by our genes and how much remains fluid, shaped by every choice we make and every thought we think? This question led me to wonder if hypnotherapy and mindset could reach beyond the subconscious mind to directly influence our very biology. Well happily, I can tell you that research, along with my own lived experience and that of many of my clients, suggests that it can.

Genetics might open our story, but it certainly doesn't write the entire script. Our thoughts, feelings, responses, and healing processes are deeply shaped by the environments we create, both externally and importantly internally.

Through focused and intentional therapeutic work, we can influence our genetic functioning and unlock our potential to create new outcomes.

For years, genes were seen as the permanent and unchanging framework of our being, shaping everything from eye colour to disease susceptibility. But now, we know that this perspective is not entirely true.

Advances in epigenetics reveal that our genes are more like a flexible framework than an unchangeable fate. Our external environment and the internal environment shaped by our thoughts, emotions, and choices profoundly influence our gene expression. Research clearly shows that factors like stress, nutrition, relationships, and even beliefs can turn genes on or off, acting like switches as they adapt to our surroundings (Goldberg et al., 2007). This understanding places us as active participants, not passive recipients, of our inherited genetic legacy.

In this context, hypnotherapy is transformative as it grants access to the subconscious, where our entrenched patterns, emotions, and inherited beliefs reside. Through gentle exploration and reframing, we can connect with this potential, opening ourselves up to new possibilities. As we do so, the body responds to create a new internal environment by creating new chemistry and promoting change on many levels.

Working in this subconscious space fosters neuroplasticity, the brain's ability to rewire itself, shedding old habits and forming healthier ones. hypnotherapy has the ability to anchor these new patterns in place with positive suggestions, visualisation, and emotional healing, leading to meaningful change.

Taking transformation further, bioplasticity refers to the dynamic adaptability of your biological systems. You see our systems are also not static models of function. Bioplasticity is demonstrated by the nervous system, and indeed the body's ability to reorganise in response to new experiences. It provides a lens for understanding how hypnotherapy may create real and lasting change. (Sanson, n.d.)

In hypnotherapy, through the process of bioplasticity, the mind's focus aligns with the body's intelligence to respond to every thought. This altered state enables changes in attention, emotional regulation, and memory consolidation reflecting bioplastic change, producing a reorganisation of the nervous system and our body's chemistry in response to internal cues.

Epigenetics, the study of how external factors influence gene expression without altering our DNA, intersects intriguingly with bioplasticity. Factors like stress, trauma, relationships, and therapy can influence genes involved in immune response, emotional regulation, and stress systems (McEwen BS., 2007). Hypnotherapy can therefore influence our genes by inducing states of deep relaxation, reducing stress, and supporting emotional integration. This results in potential epigenetic shifts, such as downregulating inflammation and supporting resilience and emotional stability.

Bioplasticity offers a new perspective on genes and our ability to heal. Bioplasticity shows us that the functioning of our genes can be influenced, and that you are not doomed to be forever the recipient of an unfortunate gene pool. Hypnotherapy can tap into this latent plasticity, reshaping both mind and biology. Change, therefore, isn't merely mental or emotional, it's cellular, influenced at the genetic level. Practices like deep relaxation, mindfulness, and affirmations common in hypnotherapy can reduce stress hormones like cortisol, which certainly has an impact on gene expression. This internal shift forms the basis of epigenetics, influencing genetic signals depending on our internal environment. (Császár, Scholkmann, & Bókkon, 2021)

When we say hypnotherapy supports change, it may be more accurate to explain that this may in part be due to the fact that hypnotherapy can influence our potential for change by affecting our biology at the genetic level. In a deep often relaxed state, the body can recalibrate. Visualisations and suggestions can affect systems such as our digestion and our immune function. In other words, this is the point where mind and body; mental and physical come together to foster holistic healing. In this harmonious state, the mind and body collaborate, allowing healing to unfold naturally.

This process creates a feedback loop that supports deep transformation, demonstrating that change isn't just possible, it's embedded in our biology, it's embedded in our genes. Epigenetics shows us this.

Our thoughts, emotions, and behaviours can regulate our gene expression. We are very aware of the effects of stress on our bodies as discussed in the previous chapter and now perhaps this begins to make more sense. We know chronic stress can activate harmful genes, while positive emotional states can up-regulate healing genes.

When we understand this powerful principle, we are open to becoming active participants in directing our biology to influence our future outcomes. Hypnotherapy, acting as a bridge between conscious and subconscious realms, can rewrite our internal narratives. As these stories shift, so does the body's responses. The mind has the ability to reframe our previous perceptions and limiting beliefs, and as it does the body obediently follows suit.

This is what I call predictable outcomes.

JODY'S STORY

Consider Jody, a 46-year-old client with chronic fatigue and IBS. She was trapped in constant alertness, emotionally depleted and carrying a subconscious belief that equated rest with laziness. Over six hypnotherapy sessions, we gently explored and released these beliefs. Jody reframed rest as necessary for healing, visualised her desired outcomes, and practiced affirmations, eventually leading to improved digestion, energy, and mood. The transformation wasn't just cognitive it was chemical. As her nervous system calmed, her body healed. This demonstrates the potential of hypnotherapy to reshape not only thoughts but also our biological internal environment.

Genes do matter, but not as rigid determinants. With hypnotherapy, leveraging neuroplasticity, bioplasticity, and epigenetic shifts, we wield an extraordinary power to influence our own well-being. We are active participants, ready to reshape our genetic futures.

The barriers that dissolve in the hypnotic state, grant us the power to reimagine not only our minds but the very fabric of our beings. Change isn't just a possibility it's our encoded human potential when we are ready and open to embrace it.

Chapter Eight

THE POWER OF FEELING – UNLOCKING THE KEY TO TRANSFORMATIONAL THERAPY

In the journey toward personal growth and healing, few things are as profound as the connection to our emotions and our feelings. Often dismissed as fleeting or intangible, feelings are in fact the language of the body that connects us to our immense human potential to transform body and mind alike.

When harnessed correctly, they create a bridge between the mind and body, stimulating and enabling deep, lasting therapeutic change. This chapter explores the importance of connecting to feeling in therapy, drawing on insights from the HeartMath Institute, the latest discoveries in neuroscience and the ongoing work of people such as Joe Dispenza, Gregg Braden and many others.

The research from the HeartMath Institute beautifully illuminates how deeply our emotions influence both our body and mind. They've discovered that the heart produces an electromagnetic field that stretches several feet beyond our physical body. A living, dynamic energy that shifts in tune with our feelings. When we experience positive emotions like gratitude, love, care or compassion, this field becomes harmonious, creating a rhythm that aligns the heart, brain, and nervous system.

Although, to the best of my knowledge, it is not discussed in the HeartMath research, I would certainly postulate that the extended neural network that we engage when in a state of heart brain coherence, would also include the gut.

Sayings like "go with your gut" or "trust your gut instinct" have stood the test of time, possibly spanning centuries, because they resonate with an inherent truth. I believe this enduring wisdom arises from the fact that the gut houses brain cells, connecting our intuitive knowing and our physical being in a profound way.

The gut is believed to have roughly 200 to 600 million neurons. Each neuron has many branches, like axons and dendrites, so the total number of these branches in the gut likely reaches billions. In contrast, according to the HeartMath Institute the heart is now understood to contain around 40,000 neurons, while the overall neurite count in the heart is estimated to be far greater than this. It therefore makes sense to me, and again I postulate, that when in the powerfully transformative state described as Heart – Brain coherence, the extended neural network would also include the neurons in the gastro-intestinal tract. Why ? Because I believe in the magnificence of the human body with all its miraculous intricacies and complexities. These neurons are present in the gut for a reason.

Research from the HeartMath institute has demonstrated that heart-brain coherence occurs when neurons in the heart and neurons in the brain are activated, forming an extended and powerful neural network. Given this, it's only natural to consider the inclusion of neurons in the gastrointestinal tract would also be a part of this comprehensive neural network

You may well ask why I discuss this in a hypnotherapy book. The reason is because I also believe this is the very same state of coherence that a person enters when in a state of hypnotic trance.

The concept of coherence, which fosters healing by creating a safe and open state, activates the parasympathetic nervous system, encouraging rest, repair, and growth. Research from HeartMath Institute indicates that achieving heart coherence not only calms us but also boosts mental clarity, ignites creativity, and enhances resilience, all of which are critical for overcoming emotional barriers.

From a neuroscience perspective, emotions can create a bridge between the subconscious mind and the body. They may arise in the limbic system, especially the amygdala, which governs our experience of fear and pleasure. Coupled with memory, emotions can weave lasting neural patterns that shape how we respond to life.

When considering this from a hypnotherapeutic perspective, we often ask our clients to imagine and connect to their desired outcome as though they have already achieved it, while connecting to all the emotions and feelings of this state. This action, often referred to as a future-pace can have the same profound neurological effects. By evoking strong emotions associated with future success, this technique engages key brain regions like the amygdala, facilitating neurotransmitter release that strengthens memory encoding. The emotional arousal aids in forming vivid lasting memories, and in the case of a Hypnotherapeutic progression, future memories, whilst enhancing synaptic plasticity, making the imagined outcomes more achievable and impactful.

Dr. Joe Dispenza sheds light on how powerful this process is in therapy. When clients deeply connect with the feeling of their desired outcome, be it peace, joy, freedom, or health, they can begin to rewire their brain's neural pathways.

As all hypnotherapists should be aware, the subconscious mind cannot tell the difference between a real event and one vividly imagined, especially when the emotions connected to the imagined outcome are felt 'as if' they are real and happening now. During therapy when we step our clients directly into their goal state and ask them to imagine vividly that they have already achieved it, they can begin to tap into the feelings of success. This isn't merely symbolic; it's an essential step towards lasting transformation because the neurological changes created help to wire this new identity firmly in place. However, this is not the full story, as we will see in the next chapter, repetition is an important and necessary component for permanent change, and the client needs to participate in the process on a daily basis for the best outcomes.

When I reflect on my own client's outcomes, it becomes apparent that those who are most invested in their own therapy by actively participating in the homework tasks allocated, are the clients who have the best outcomes and go on to achieve their desired goals.

As Dispenza so eloquently states, "When you embody elevated emotions like gratitude or love, or health, you're telling your body the experience you seek has already happened." This embodiment, or future pace as hypnotherapists may call it, has the potential to fast-track healing, with the body naturally mirroring and responding to the mind's new neurological, biological or genetic blueprint.

So, if we agree that emotions speak to the body in a language the body and the subconscious mind both understand and respond to, and they certainly do, then I believe hypnosis is the doorway through which we may access that ability to communicate most directly. While our conscious mind often holds tightly to logic and judgement, hypnosis creates a more receptive state where emotions can be felt fully and authentically, without the interference from our conscious mind. This immersive experience enables clients to connect to their emotions, whilst moving beyond any intellectual limitations as they pave the way forward for profound change and optimal outcomes.

As mentioned in the chapter on the brain, when a client enters hypnosis, the usual mental filters soften, and the emotional heart rhythm can shift toward coherence, much like the states HeartMath research highlights. As a HeartMath practitioner and a very experienced Clinical hypnotherapist, it is my absolute belief that our clients enter a state of heart brain coherence during hypnosis. This calm, harmonious state, leads the nervous system to switch from Sympathetic nervous system activation:

fight-flight- freeze mode to parasympathetic nervous system activation: rest-and-repair mode, providing fertile ground for healing. Hypnosis doesn't just create positive feelings it can amplify them, helping clients to embody sensations like safety, love, confidence, or calm to name but a few, in a way that feels real and accessible in the present moment.

To summarise, the emotional engagement during hypnosis creates a powerful rewiring of neural pathways. Through guided imagery, suggestion, somatic awareness and a curious exploration of possible outcomes, hypnosis helps the client feel the future they desire in the present moment. Seeds are planted for new patterns of thought, emotion, and behaviour to take root. With repetition, the importance of which will be further discussed in the next chapter, the subconscious mind responds as though the imagined scenario is now real. This leads to different thoughts and different feelings becoming the new normal, as the process of neural rewiring accommodates and strengthens the desired outcomes. In this way, hypnosis can become a unique experiential bridge which connects mind and body through the deep current of emotion and feelings. It's here that true healing begins, not as an abstract concept, but as a living, embodied reality supported by our magnificent physiology: mind-brain-body.

EMMA'S JOURNEY

Consider 'Emma,' a client struggling with overwhelming anxiety that left her feeling trapped in a cycle of fear and exhaustion. Despite knowing logically that her fears weren't grounded in present reality, the emotional charge was so intense that it hijacked her nervous system daily.

Utilising hypnosis, Emma was gently guided into a state of deep relaxation where her usual mental chatter quietened, and her subconscious mind became more accessible. In this receptive space, she was able to connect with feelings of safety and calm, emotions that had long been elusive and previously overshadowed by anxiety.

Using imagery of a peaceful, safe place and hypnotic suggestions tailored specifically to her goal state, Emma was able to embody a sense of being grounded and resilient. As her mind and body became more coherent with each therapy session, and each daily homework session attended, Emma's nervous system began to shift out of a state of hyperarousal and move towards a state of calm.

This wasn't just a mental exercise for Emma; it was a profound emotional experience that aided in rewiring her brain's neurology and her bodies biology every time she experienced the peaceful and importantly safe state.

Over several sessions, and a lot of essential practice outside the therapy room, through self-hypnotic techniques, and conscious interruption of old habits and patterns, the new feelings of safety became more accessible outside of hypnosis. Emma was instructed to monitor her self-talk, interrupt outdated negative patterns and to look for the changes that were occurring daily. She was instructed to notice her ability to experience situations in the way she had vividly felt and imagined she could. This helped Emma to create and neurologically rewire a different, more acceptable response to stressful situations.

This embodied emotional shift changed the story her body was telling her. What once felt like an unshakeable state of anxiety gradually transformed into a lived experience of peace and resilience enabling her to deal with life's daily stressors. By working deeply with her emotional feelings and previously automatic unhelpful responses, Emma was able to redirect her internal physiology and biology, effectively opening the door to lasting healing.

Hypnosis is far more than a tool for soothing distress or managing difficult emotions. Its true power shines brightest when the same focus and energy that once fed the problem are intentionally redirected toward the solution. In this shift of attention, something remarkable happens: the body begins to respond to a completely new set of instructions.

We want our clients like Emma to purposely shift from dwelling on fear, pain, or limitation to vividly experiencing and imagining hope, confidence, or healing. Hypnosis can deepen that experience in a way that feels immediate and tangible. As stated, the subconscious mind doesn't separate imagination from reality. It receives these fresh signals and starts to rewrite old patterns. The body follows, adapting its physiological responses to align with this new narrative.

For example, rather than reinforcing anxiety and overwhelm through focus on old limiting thoughts feelings and emotions, the nervous system learns to settle into calm instead of sitting in an imagined anxiety. Instead of triggering inflammation, it embraces restoration. This rewiring opens a space where possibilities replace barriers, and resilience can grow stronger with each session. The client doesn't just think differently, they act, respond and live differently, therefore embodying a renewed sense of self that supports sustained wellbeing.

This is where the profound potential for hypnotherapeutic transmutation occurs: by harnessing the body's innate capacity to mirror the mind's new blueprint, healing moves beyond relief toward transformation. The journey is not merely about easing symptoms but awakening the body's natural wisdom to thrive.

Let's expand this concept beyond the confines of therapy into the vast realm of consciousness. Gregg Braden, an influential figure at the crossroads of science and spirituality, presents an intriguing viewpoint: emotions transcend mere internal states; they act as energetic currents that engage with the external world. By integrating ancient wisdom with new scientific insights, Braden proposes that emotions are potent architects of reality, emitting signals that influence the events, connections, and the possibilities we draw into our lives.

This idea has profound implications in therapy. When we help a client connect with the feeling of the life they long to live be it joy, peace, confidence, love or abundance, we're not just helping them imagine change; we're helping them embody it. In doing so, they begin to emit a different energetic frequency. And, according to Braden, that emotional signal becomes a kind of instruction to the quantum field, an invitation for life to respond in kind.

Let me be clear, this is not about magical thinking or bypassing life's challenges. It's about aligning the client's internal state: thoughts, feelings, and beliefs, so fully with their desired future that they become a living expression of it.

As Braden beautifully puts it, "Feeling is the prayer." When intention and emotion are fused, the field of possibility opens, and change begins to ripple outward, not only within the client, but in the world that surrounds them.

Direct connection between emotions and the quantum field remains speculative in mainstream science, however from a clinical perspective, this speculative energetic connection between emotion and the quantum field offers a powerful framework for understanding how deep change unfolds in therapy. When a client steps into the feeling of their desired outcome during hypnosis or guided imagery, they are essentially rehearsing a new way of being, not just in their mind, but at a cellular and energetic level. Hypnosis becomes the vehicle through which this journey may occur.

Take for example, the case of 'James.' A man struggling with chronic pain that had resisted conventional treatment. Through hypnosis, James' focus was directed toward noticing relief by discovering and connecting to a profound sense of comfort. He experienced emotions he hadn't accessed in years. James' shift wasn't purely superficial; it served to activate new neural pathways which could lead to an alteration in his body's stress response. Thus, allowing his physiology to begin the healing process, which would significantly impact his biology in positive ways. A reminder of what we already know: when feelings are truly embraced, as shown through the extensive research of the HeartMath institute, our internal chemistry is significantly changed.

They have shown that activating a renewing emotion, such as gratitude or compassion and holding it for as little as three minutes, can lead to these positive changes being measurable in the body for up to six hours.

Clinically, this reveals something essential. It is not enough for our clients to simply acknowledge what is wrong, true healing requires that the client believe and embody what is possible. By fostering this embodied experience through hypnotherapy, a clear signal is received, not only by the subconscious mind but by the broader energetic systems of the body, that a different reality is both imaginable and attainable.

This insight reminds us that healing is not linear. It moves in waves, sparked by the client's capacity to truly feel into their future self with conviction. Self- doubt will just as quickly allow for the forward movement to often circle back around. As in the words of Henry Ford who once famously said, "Whether you think you can, or you think you can't, you're right." This quote underscores the powerful role of mindset in determining one's success or failure. In such situations, hypnosis can become the vessel that carries intention and emotional feelings into the deepest layers of our being, directly to where transformation can occur.

As a certified HeartMath® practitioner with many years of experience, as well as a seasoned tutor and practitioner of clinical hypnotherapy, I hold a strong conviction that truly effective therapy depends on bringing the heart and brain into harmonious coherence. This is not merely a poetic idea; it is grounded in research and biology. The heart produces an electromagnetic field thousands of times stronger than that of the brain, making it a powerful influence on our emotional and physiological states. When clients learn to tune into their heart's intelligence, they can access a deeper, more intuitive form of knowing.

In summary, and while more research is needed, I firmly believe that during a deep hypnotic state, clients naturally enter a state of heart-brain coherence. This process involves more than simply thinking about desired outcomes; it requires actually feeling them as though they have already been realised. This is where hypnosis reveals its true potential, allowing us to gently guide clients to 'future pace' themselves into the very state they wish to embody.

Self-hypnosis offers an incredibly empowering tool for clients to deepen and extend the therapeutic work beyond the clinical setting. One of its greatest strengths lies in its ability to allow the clients to connect to the feelings and emotions of their desired state. It also harnesses the brain's natural capacity for neural repetition, an essential process for awakening and rewiring neural pathways that support lasting change.

When we experience something repeatedly, the brain strengthens the connections that encode those experiences into lasting habits, beliefs, and emotional responses. Self-hypnosis provides a structured, accessible way for clients to practise this repetition intentionally, engaging the subconscious mind in a focused and relaxed state. This is where true transformation begins to take root.

By regularly guiding themselves into trance, connecting to positive emotions and reinforcing positive suggestions or visualisations, clients effectively retrain their brains to align with their desired outcomes, whether that's greater confidence, relief from pain, or emotional resilience. The repetitive nature of self-hypnosis helps bypass the critical, analytical conscious mind, allowing new patterns to be absorbed deeply and organically.

Beyond rewiring neural circuits, self-hypnosis fosters a sense of agency and self-trust. Clients learn to become active participants in their own healing journey, developing tools to access calm, clarity, and inner wisdom whenever needed. This ongoing practice cultivates a positive feedback loop: as clients experience shifts and successes, their motivation to continue deepens, further reinforcing the new neural pathways.

Ultimately, self-hypnosis, which we will talk more about in the next chapter empowers the 'client' to create change in a controlled and sustainable way, not just having to rely on a one-time event in a clinical setting.

Practical techniques like HeartMath's Quick Coherence® exercise are also invaluable tools to enhance therapeutic outcomes in the client process throughout the waking state. By focusing on the heart, regulating breathing, and consciously evoking positive feelings, clients can shift from stress to calmness in seconds. This shift lays the foundation for deeper therapeutic work, as the client becomes more present, receptive, and aligned with their inner wisdom and once again connecting to feeling is a pivotal part of this process.

Therapy often focuses on cognition: understanding thoughts, analysing patterns, and reframing beliefs. While this is naturally very important, it's only part of the equation. I believe true transformation occurs when intellect converges with the power of feeling.

Science tells us feelings are the catalyst for change because they engage the subconscious mind, the body, and the quantum field simultaneously. When clients connect deeply to the feeling of being healed, empowered, or free, they can often transcend the limitations of their current circumstances due to the immediate responses of their physiology and biology, as discussed.

As therapists, our role is to guide clients into the emotional state that aligns with their goals. This requires creating a safe coherent space and encouraging clients to envision and embody their desired outcomes with emotional intensity. We have the privilege and responsibility of helping our clients connect to their deepest emotions, unlocking their inner power, and creating a reality that reflects their highest potential.

In the words of Joe Dispenza, "To change your personal reality, you must change your personality." This involves stepping into a new state of being, and the gateway to that state is feeling. Whether through hypnosis and self-hypnosis, hypnotic guided visualisation, somatic practices, or HeartMath techniques, I believe that our ability to connect to the feeling of something greater than the now, is the cornerstone of effective therapy.

By integrating insights from the latest research in therapeutic hypnosis, neuroscience and HeartMath® interventions, or by tuning into the wisdom of visionaries like Joe Dispenza and Gregg Braden and many others, we can create a therapeutic experience for our clients that empowers them to transform from the inside out.

Feeling is not just a byproduct of change, I believe it is the very mechanism through which change occurs.

Chapter Nine

UNLOCKING CHANGE: THE IMPACT OF SELF-HYPNOSIS AND REPETITION

Self-hypnosis is a powerful technique that enables individuals to access their subconscious mind and bring about meaningful shifts in their thoughts, feelings, and behaviours. Unlike guided hypnotherapy sessions led by a professional, self-hypnosis empowers people to take charge of their own healing process. With regular practice, it can help foster relaxation, alleviate stress, overcome limiting beliefs, and strengthen positive habits.

As briefly mentioned in the previous chapter, I believe the key to effective self-hypnosis lies in repetition. Like acquiring any new skill, be it learning a musical instrument or improving athletic ability, consistent practice is essential. Practice in this instance involves repeatedly reinforcing positive suggestions, which helps to rewire the brain's neural pathways, making lasting change more achievable and sustainable.

What Is Self-Hypnosis?

Self-hypnosis involves guiding oneself into a focused, often relaxed subconscious state, allowing access to the deeper, creative and less judgemental part of the mind. In this state, the mind becomes more receptive to suggestions, allowing individuals to address deeply ingrained patterns or beliefs that may be keeping them stuck in problematic thinking, feeling or behaviours.

Often utilised to achieve a deeply relaxed state, self-hypnosis offers so much more than that. it becomes a gentle, yet powerful invitation to step away from our problems into the deeper wisdom of the subconscious mind, and in doing so connect to our desired solutions and resourced states.

Through self-hypnosis, we can often identify clear goals and the necessary changes we or our clients wish to achieve. In this powerfully transformative state, we also have the ability to begin to cultivate sharper focus and unlock our creative potential, whilst strengthening our emotional resilience. Limiting beliefs can gently dissipate and be replaced with more beneficial ones that uplift and empower the recipient. All of which can help us navigate life's challenges with greater ease and foresight.

Unlike meditation, which lovingly invites us to rest in awareness and presence, self-hypnosis carries an intentionality to embark on a purposeful journey towards meaningful transformation.

Like all lasting change, be it the goal to build muscles from gym work outs or training to successfully complete a marathon, I believe repetition is the cornerstone to success. Self-hypnosis is no different. The subconscious mind learns through repeated exposure, much like the way a path becomes clear and defined after being walked many times. With each repetition, the brain strengthens neural connections associated with the desired outcome or belief, gradually shifting these patterns from intentional practice to automatic behaviour.

Neuroscience demonstrates that repetition reinforces neural pathways through a process known as neuroplasticity (Doidge, 2007). When positive suggestions are repeated during self-hypnosis, and desired outcomes are experienced in real time by the recipients, new neural circuits are created that replace the unhelpful ones which have been running outdated patterns and habits. Over time, these circuits become the brain's default mode of thinking, feeling and responding.

The subconscious mind can often resist change, especially when deeply ingrained beliefs or habits are involved. This is why regular practice is so important as it helps bypass this resistance. With each session, the subconscious becomes more familiar with and more accepting of the new suggestion, integrating them more seamlessly into everyday life.

The repetition possible with self-hypnotic client homework ensures that the work done in the session is reinforced at home, allowing the ongoing benefits of the therapeutic session to become more permanent.

Although one hypnosis session can often bring quick relief and sincere moments of clarity, lasting change is most often accompanied by regular practice. Think back to the section on neural plasticity. It's all about a mind and body shift. When we do something different or when we believe something different, we become something different.

Again, back to our gym analogy, you don't do a single sit-up and suddenly have a six-pack. It's the steady commitment and repetition that truly sculpt the results. So, if you want a mind that's fit and fabulous, you had better get ready to show up more than once. There are no shortcuts to brain abs here!

So how do we create a practice that works?

The first important step is to create a clear intention. What are you hoping to achieve, and when and how are you intending to achieve it? You might begin by identifying a specific goal or area for improvement. This could be reducing anxiety, improving sleep, or building confidence.

We then need to find a quiet, comfortable space where you won't be disturbed. It is sometimes beneficial to choose the same location as the brain may begin to associate this space with tranquillity and almost act as a positional anchor to assist you entering a hypnotic state easily and effectively.

When you have found your self-hypnosis space, begin with turning your focus of attention inward. Slowing the breath, enabling it to be slightly longer and deeper than usual, paying particular attention to the out breath allowing it to lengthen even more as you relax into each long, slow exhalation. Sometimes a progressive muscle relaxation can be utilised to calm the body and quiet the mind. When done correctly, all of this brings us into a coherent state of calm as we simultaneously activate our parasympathetic nervous system.

Once in a deep state of focused attention, a specific image, word, or sensation that aligns with your intention may be recalled. Images or preferred responses must always be framed or imagined in the present tense, 'as-if-now', utilising solution focused or positive language only. For instance, instead of saying, "I won't be feeling anxious," say instead something like, "I am calm and in control." Affirmations to be used during self-hypnosis are also crafted in the same way, as if you have already achieved them.

Allow your mind to create a state of knowing what this will be like. Please remember however you do this is just fine. As we are all individuals, there is no right or wrong here. Some may imagine this as a vision, others may hear words of affirmation from themself or from others, and many others will just get a sense of feeling it. However you do it, imagine it as though you have already achieved it and allow yourself to really lean into the feelings of your desired state. Repeat this activity again and again.

Commit to your self-hypnosis practice daily, even if only for a few minutes, it will generally culminate in leading you to your desired outcomes sooner. Let's not forget, repetition strengthens neuroplasticity and the body's physiological and psychological response to the suggestions.

JANE'S JOURNEY

Jane, a 45-year-old business owner, is a good example of the power of repetition. Jane came to the clinic to manage her stress and improve her sleep. Initially sceptical, she committed to practicing self-hypnosis for 10 minutes every evening. Her affirmations focused on calm and rest: "My mind and body are relaxed and calm", "I easily drift into a deep, restorative sleep." "I sleep soundly and peacefully every night." "I wake up feeling refreshed, rested and ready for the new day." "I maintain a feeling of calm when at work."

During her self-hypnosis sessions, Jane let her subconscious mind fully embrace each affirmation by fully immersing herself in her imagination and embodying them experientially.

In the first week, Jane found it challenging to quieten her mind, but she persisted. By the second week, she noticed subtle changes, her racing thoughts slowed, and she began falling asleep more easily.

After one month of daily practice, Jane could notice many changes which drove her to diligently continue her practice. By six weeks of daily practice Jane reported being able to achieve a deeper, more restful sleep and an improved ability to handle stress during her workday.

She credited her progress to the consistency of her practice and stated her intention to continue. The continuation of Jane's daily practice was an important point of discussion. Not just for Jane, but for all of our clients and indeed ourselves. So many people conscientiously do the assigned practices, working with the therapeutic tools given and achieve wonderful states of success, subsequently reporting feeling so much better, however this can often be the trap. When people feel better, they may be tempted to stop doing the self-care or therapeutic practices that have allowed them to feel better in the first place. It is no surprise therefore that when this happens, our old habits and patterns of thinking and feeling may begin to slip back into play. Unfortunately, clients may then be disappointed to discover that their problems have returned.

Once again if we use the gym analogy: you go to gym, you do the repetitions to build those spectacular muscles and sculpt that body of your dreams, however when you stop doing the work you may find the 'old you' looking back at you in the mirror in the morning.

In the words of that old, yet oh so familiar saying, "if you don't use it, you lose it."

Studies indicate that self-hypnosis effectively alleviates stress, anxiety, and chronic pain. Hammond's 2010 research revealed substantial enhancements in both physical and emotional health among those who consistently practiced self-hypnosis. A crucial element in achieving these benefits was the frequent and repetitious application of positive suggestions. Research on neuroplasticity also highlights the significance of repetition in effecting enduring changes within the brain. Doidge (2007) illustrates how continual mental practice can transform and reshape neural pathways, resonating with the concepts of self-hypnosis.

I have my own ideas about the necessity for repetition to enhance beneficial therapeutic outcomes. As a clinical hypnotherapist and counsellor, I emphasise the importance of awareness and repetition in my practice. I encourage my clients to be aware of repetitive outdated habits and patterns, and how to interrupt these limiting processes, redirecting their focus to their desired outcomes. The integration of self-hypnosis and keeping their focus on their desired outcomes by integrating these practices into their daily routines is pivotal in weakening old neural pathways as new ones are strengthened. I often compare the process to nurturing and caring for a beautiful garden, removing the intruders one weed at a time. The more consistently you tend to it, the stronger and healthier it grows.

Self-hypnosis is an empowering and transformative practice that allows individuals to take charge of their mental and emotional well-being. I believe its success lies not only in the method but also in the consistency of applying positive suggestions through repetition. The role repetition plays is pivotal in overcoming previously ingrained habits and patterns. For many clients, the first few sessions of self-hypnosis may feel unfamiliar or even ineffective. However, by trusting the process and committing to regular practice, they often settle into a familiarity of the exercise which can open themselves up to experience profound shifts. The strengthening of new neural pathways, that accompanies regular self-hypnosis helps to overcome resistance and can lead to the creation of lasting change. In this process repetition becomes foundational for success, personal growth and healing.

Whether you or your client's goal is to reduce stress, build confidence, or break free from limiting beliefs, self-hypnosis offers a practical and accessible path to transformation, one intentional session at a time.

Chapter Ten

THE ROLE OF SUGGESTION

Central to the practice of hypnotherapy is the concept of suggestion, a powerful therapeutic tool that significantly influences the subconscious mind. This chapter explores the vital role of suggestion in hypnotherapy, examining its mechanisms, types, applications, and the scientific principles that underpin its effectiveness. By understanding how suggestion operates, practitioners and clients alike can appreciate its capacity to facilitate profound change.

As all well-trained clinical hypnotherapists will know, the use of suggestion in hypnotherapy carries important ethical responsibilities. Hypnotherapists must always prioritise the client's well-being and autonomy, proceeding only after informed consent.

Every hypnotherapist understands that a client remains in complete control while in a trance and can exit this state at any time if they choose not to accept a given suggestion. Nonetheless, suggestions should never be crafted to manipulate or coerce clients into actions that conflict with their values or desires. The purpose and nature of the suggestions our clients receive with regard to the direction and goal of the therapeutic session should be discussed and agreed upon prior to trance enabling clients to participate actively in their healing process.

In hypnotherapy, suggestion entails introducing goal-oriented ideas, beliefs, or instructions to the subconscious mind in a way that promotes acceptance and integration. Unlike the conscious mind, which tends to be analytical and often resistant to change, the subconscious operates with fewer filters, bypassing critical judgment and making it highly receptive to therapeutic interventions.

During a typical hypnotic state, clients often experience a heightened focus of attention, often but not always, associated with relaxation. This state creates an ideal environment for therapeutic suggestions to be received and accepted, a term sometimes referred to as enhanced suggestibility. In this altered state hypnotherapists seek to provide suggestions which can bypass the critical, often sceptical conscious mind, and therefore connect directly with the subconscious. It is essential to emphasise that suggestion is not about control or coercion; rather, hypnotherapy is a collaborative process where well-constructed suggestions align with the client's values and willingness to change. If a client is unwilling to change, no amount of well-constructed and carefully delivered suggestions will be effective.

Clinical hypnotherapists are well trained in the construction of various types of suggestions, each tailored to meet the unique needs of their individual clients. Deciding which type of suggestion and the preferred delivery for the individual client you are working with can sometimes be the definitive factor that can enhance both the effectiveness of the therapeutic process and the client's experience:

Direct Suggestions:

Direct suggestions are clear, explicit instructions designed to communicate with the subconscious mind. These suggestions are particularly effective for addressing specific issues and are most impactful when formulated using the client's solution-focused language, typically expressed positively and in the present tense, as if it is happening now. By doing so, these suggestions promote integration, allowing the client to vividly imagine and connect with their desired solution or goal state. For instance, a therapist might say, "You feel confident and comfortable in social situations." Or "You wake up feeling rested, energised and ready for your day after a good night's sleep."

Indirect Suggestions:

Indirect suggestions foster self-discovery and can facilitate profound psychological shifts leading to sustainable change and personal growth. They are more subtle than direct suggestion and are often conveyed through the use of metaphors or vague statements, allowing the subconscious mind to interpret the meaning personally. Milton Erickson was well known for his effective use of indirect suggestions which engaged clients who may otherwise have been analytical or dubious as to the process. In such instances indirect suggestion can be effectively used to bypass these cognitive resistances. An example of an indirect suggestion could be "You may find that as you relax more and more you can discover a different kind of feeling in all those situations" or "As you reflect on your strengths you can notice so many things are changing in just the way you imagined they might"

Embedded Suggestions:

These suggestions are phrases woven into or disguised within larger narratives. The intention is to capture the subconscious's attention through subtle emphasis of particular words. For instance, a hypnotherapist may say, "No matter where you are you can use what you've learned to *release muscular tightness with each exhalation*, and you may be curious to discover how easy it is for you to... *create an enduring sense of calm.*" This technique is a key component of conversational hypnosis as it subtly guides clients without direct instructions.

Post-Hypnotic Suggestions:

Post-hypnotic suggestions are suggestions given as directives during a hypnotic state which are intended to take effect after the session. An example would be, "Every day as you notice more and more positive changes are happening you feel motivated to continue making healthy choices." These suggestions play a vital role in enhancing therapeutic results, ensuring that the advantages of hypnotherapy session continue beyond the appointment.

Metaphorical Suggestions:

A metaphorical suggestion is a form of hypnotic suggestion that uses imagery or symbolic language to facilitate deeper understanding, stimulate personal responses and facilitate change. This approach uses metaphors, imagery or story to convey deeper meanings. The aim is that clients will relate and respond to the concepts on a personal level. Metaphorical suggestions encourage clients to explore their own thoughts and feelings, encouraging insight and personal transformation in a more natural and resonant manner. An example of a metaphoric suggestion is "Even as the storm continues to rage, it is possible to guide the ship into the shelter of a protected cove finding protection until the storm passes, as all storms eventually do"

Confusion suggestion:

Confusional suggestions or technique, is often employed to deliberately create ambiguity or uncertainty. It can be utilised to bypass the client's critical thinking processes or resistances. By suggesting contradictory or overly complex scenarios the hypnotherapist encourages the conscious mind to tire and the subconscious mind to take charge enabling deeper access to thoughts, emotions, and resources. This approach can help overly analytical clients let go of resistance, facilitating change by allowing them to explore new perspectives and insights without the interference of analytical thinking.

Paradoxical suggestion:

Paradoxical suggestion involves inviting the client to do the opposite of what they consciously want to achieve in order to reduce its power or change its pattern. This is a subtle, often underestimated tool in clinical hypnotherapy. At first glance it appears to contradict the client's goals, yet it can be remarkably effective in the hands of a skilled practitioner.

The paradox bypasses resistance as it speaks directly to the subconscious mind, and this is where real healing can take root. We see it often with sleep issues. A client who suffers insomnia might be given a surprising suggestion: for example- "Tonight, see how long you can keep yourself awake, really try."

This gentle reversal interrupts the anxious effort to force sleep that inadvertently fuels insomnia. Effectively removing the pressure to sleep makes way for the natural process of sleep to be restored. What's really unfolding here is the paradox offers the client permission to stop struggling with themselves. In that permission, inner conflict can begin to dissolve.

This technique aligns closely with the work of Milton Erickson, who taught that indirect suggestion, utilisation, and creative engagement with the subconscious mind are often more powerful than direct instruction. Likewise, Viktor Frankl employed what he called "paradoxical intention" to help clients confront, or invite, their most feared symptoms, thus robbing them of their power.

When applied ethically and with clinical discernment, paradoxical suggestion has the potential to disrupt entrenched patterns and facilitate meaningful therapeutic change, particularly in cases where conventional strategies prove ineffective. Rather than opposing resistance, the therapist engages with it strategically, transforming it into a vehicle for insight and growth.

Utilisation as Suggestion:

At the heart of effective hypnotherapy lies a relatively simple concept: utilisation.

This is a concept that invites the therapist to work with what is available within the client's reality, their internal experience and the external world. Their language, beliefs, experiences, and even their resistances can all be skilfully used to deepen trance and act as convincers. Outside noises or occurrences that may otherwise be a distraction can also be utilised to deepen the client's inner experience. It is an approach grounded in respect for the client's inner world and trust in the subconscious mind's capacity to reorganise, reframe and heal.

The process of utilisation may begin with the hypnotherapist noticing something as subtle as an involuntary muscle release, or an emotion that begins to surface within a session, as we acknowledge and allow these things using phrases such as 'that's right you can release all of that and more.' Metaphors the client automatically uses can be utilised by incorporating them into the trance state, creating acceptance and rapport to further enhance therapy. Likewise outside distractions such as the sound of a car driving down the street to a distant destination can be utilised to remind the client that life is a lot like that car, as you move on your own journey from where you have been to your preferred destination, and like the car you can get there at your own perfect pace. Utilisation may also involve a recalled image, a physical sensation, or even the client's breathing pattern when discussing something significant. In hypnosis, these aspects serve as essential components for crafting suggestions. Instead of steering the client away from their present experience, the therapist incorporates this into the session to achieve a desired goal.

Dr Milton Erickson was very well known for his ability to work with and utilise whatever the client brought into the room. He believed that each client possessed the resources they required for their own healing journey. The therapist's role was to help them find their own resources, not to present external solutions.

Utilisation continues to be an invaluable technique within the therapist's toolkit. Take, for instance, a client who faces persistent intrusive thoughts during their hypnotherapy session. Initially, seen as a frustrating distraction, the same thoughts can be utilised with suggestions such as: "As you notice how those thoughts can go just as quickly as they came, you can get curious just how relaxing it can be to let go now" or " You may notice how every thought you release relaxes you even more" What was previously viewed as a hindrance transforms into a supportive ally in the therapeutic journey.

External distractions, such as a ticking clock can be utilised to bring the client into the present moment. An unexpected knock at the door can be utilised to represent opportunity knocking or utilised as a suggestion of opportunity – "as one door closes another is calling to you to open", distant siren, or a barking dog " and as the world busily continues on around you it can be so comforting to know there is nothing you need to do right now – except relax even more."

These suggestions allow for all things to be incorporated into the client session and put to good use. It is part of a philosophy that reflects the belief that all things the client brings to the session can be powerfully utilised in suggestions that are readily accepted by the client. As hypnotherapists I urge you to become very skilled at the practice of utilisation.

Double bind suggestions:

Double bind suggestions are powerful techniques often used by hypnotherapists. They create a scenario whereby the client is presented with two or more choices for action. Designed to empower the client to feel they are active in choosing their path forward. Double binds should be constructed using a positive focus, ensuring both options are equally appealing to the client. They generally also encourage client curiosity and exploration.

When constructing a good double bind, the hypnotherapists must first discover what change is desired by the client. The therapist then creates generally two suggestions both of which lead the individual toward their desired goal. Indirect language works well here as it further allows the suggestion to bypass the critical mind.

An example of a well-constructed double bind for a child reluctant to clean their room due to other more pleasing options could be; "I know how important playing cricket with Bob after school is to you, so perhaps you could consider either cleaning your room before school, or you could do it as soon as you get home, so you can really enjoy your time with Bob uninterrupted"

The inference is that either way the child will clean the room and still get to do what is important to him. You may also notice the rapport building and subsequent suggestions are benefitting the client whilst also pleasing Mum and achieving the desired outcome creating peace in the household.

or

For the reluctant student: "As you think about finishing your Uni assignment, you can remember how it feels to have achieved something special in the past, and in doing so you can begin to feel more motivated to give this your full attention today or perhaps you may feel just as excited to discover that taking things more slowly by doing an hour each day this week will also get you to the desired outcome."

~

The effectiveness of suggestion in hypnotherapy is linked to the interaction between the subconscious mind and neuroplasticity; the brain's capacity to reorganise itself by forming new neural connections. Neuroplasticity is enhanced whilst in a state of trance, as mentioned in previous chapters. When a suggestion is accepted by the subconscious, it can strengthen neural pathways related to desired behaviours or beliefs. For instance, a suggestion to feel calm in stressful situations may initially require conscious effort but through ongoing repetition, it can become an automatic reaction (Hammond, 1990). Here we also see the very important principle of repetition having its impact.

As mentioned in the previous chapter, a client's ability to embody or connect to the emotion of the suggestion also plays a significant role in its efficacy. Suggestions that evoke positive feelings, such as hope, joy, gratitude or relief, are more likely to be embraced and acted upon by the client. This emotional connection has the potential to amplify the suggestion's impact, embedding it more deeply in the subconscious.

Suggestions are frequently employed to assist clients in modifying habits, whether it's quitting smoking, reducing anxiety or depression or adopting healthier lifestyles. For example, the suggestion, "Each time you feel anxious, you immediately take a long, slow exhalation and feel a wave of calm and confidence filtering through you" empowers clients to replace unhealthy thought patterns with positive alternatives.

Many research articles have supported the benefit of hypnotic suggestions in altering the perception of pain. Phrases such as, "Your body feels cool and comfortable in the area where you used to feel discomfort" reframes the familiar words used to describe the experience of 'pain' that the subconscious mind knows so well. In this example the word pain is changed to 'discomfort' which alters how the brain interprets this information, signalling the body to respond differently, providing relief without the need for medication (Jensen & Patterson, 2014).

At this point it is important to remember what we have previously said regarding what we focus on we amplify. Thus, if we go looking for pain we will most certainly find it however, the converse also applies. Look for something else and expect to find it and you may be pleasantly surprised. This will be discussed further in Chapter 19. Hypnotherapy for Pain Management.

Suggestions can address emotional wounds linked to trauma, anxiety, or depression. For instance, "Now you are safe and supported, you can enjoy the feeling of letting go of the things from the past you no longer need to hold," aids clients in reframing their painful experiences as being in the past and fosters resilience in the present.

Hypnotherapy can enhance performance and self-assurance, be it in sports, public speaking, or creative endeavours. Using carefully crafted suggestions we can help our clients with a variety of presenting concerns, which will be discussed in subsequent chapters of this book. In doing so, we guide our clients as they embark on their own journey of discovering lasting change.

I'm confident that most hypnotherapists have, at some point, utilised suggestions embedded in generic scripts, which can be valuable during the learning process. However, for those more experienced in the field, I would advise caution against relying on this practice as a general rule of thumb. Suggestions are most effective when they are specifically tailored to the individual client, addressing their unique needs, desires, and goals. This personalised approach enhances the success of the hypnotherapeutic process and promotes positive change.

The versatility of suggestion stands as a cornerstone of hypnotherapeutic practice, adaptable to a range of issues and goals such as behavioural changes and physical and emotional concerns. Becoming adept at this essential element is paramount to mastering the practice of hypnotherapy. By truly listening to our clients, really hearing their words, and tailoring them in very specific, often subtle ways that resonate with their subconscious minds, we can often bypass resistances. In this way our clients subconscious mind more readily embraces these suggestions not merely as pleasant notions but as wholly attainable realities.

As we look toward the future, advancements in neuroscience and psychological research are shedding light on the mechanisms of suggestion, illuminating the way forward for more targeted and effective applications. Neuroimaging studies have explored how the brain responds to suggestions and adaptively reorganises in response to new information (Kelly & Garavan, 2005). In this evolving landscape, hypnotherapy is poised to become a more integral aspect of healthcare. Recognised not merely as a niche practice but as a versatile, evidence-based tool for healing and personal growth.

The future of hypnotherapy is not just about the introduction of new techniques; it represents a fundamental shift in our understanding of the human mind, its mechanisms and responses. With this understanding we are encouraged to recognise that very often healing comes from within. With hypnotherapy, I believe we hold the key to unlocking the gift of our human potential, paving the way forward into an era where the integration of mind and body practices can very often lead to holistic well-being.

Chapter Eleven

THE LANGUAGE OF TRANSFORMATION: METAPHOR AND STORY IN HYPNOTHERAPY

In the realm of the hypnotherapy clinic, stories and metaphors serve as the gentle often colourful brushstrokes on the canvas of the mind, or the colourful stitches of a tapestry that are unveiled one by one to reveal Images that illuminate the bigger picture, creating emotions that often words alone cannot capture. Just as any skilled artist layers paint to evoke depth and resonance, a hypnotherapist's tools are story and symbolic language that are weaved into tales of possibility, used to guide our clients on a journey of self-discovery and transformation.

These narratives are not mere embellishments; they represent the keys that unlock the subconscious mind, opening doors to memories, emotions, and insights long buried beneath the surface.

The beauty of metaphor and story lies in its ability to bypass the logical gatekeeper, as it speaks directly to the inner knowing of our clients, directly to their heart and soul, and in doing so, a path forward is carved, succeeding where previous logic has failed. This happens as a result of the subconscious becoming more accessible and open to suggestion. In this altered state, a story transforms into an experience.

An important point to remember; we know the subconscious mind doesn't differentiate between real and imagined events; it therefore responds as the story unfolds in real-time. When a client envisions climbing a mountain and reaching the summit, they experience the exhilaration of accomplishment as though they had just achieved it. This is why sensory detail is crucial in therapeutic storytelling.

The more vividly a story is told, the more immersive it becomes. However, we must also be careful with our detail so as not to take our client down a rocky dirt path when they are already halfway down and ancient set of steps.

Detail is important, but you may prefer to allow the client to fill in the gaps themselves through skilfully designed indirect suggestion, such as "you may notice the surface underneath your feet and how it feels and sounds to take each step." Or rather than being specific you can take your client into a beautiful garden and ask them to notice the trees. However, if you then ask them to smell the scent of pine trees, and they are in an English garden you will break rapport. Equally, if you have them floating gracefully in the ocean so that all their cares can wash right off them with the gentle lapping of the blue cooling waters, and they happen to be afraid of drowning or of sharks, your desired effect will be far from being achieved. We can engage all the senses to create a rich, resonant experience for our clients, but please always let it be their experience, not yours.

As we delve further into this chapter, let us explore the artful dance of story and symbolism in hypnotherapy; the playing field where imagination converges with physiology and neurology to foster healing and transformation as a story waits to unfold. This transformation may begin, as many stories do, with a single 'ah ha' moment of realisation, change, or perhaps in surrender to an inner knowing that has been lying deep beneath the surface. In the world of hypnotherapy, this pivotal moment serves as the seed hidden within well-constructed symbolism, sewn into the fertile soil of the client's mind in which that seed grows roots.

Metaphors and stories are more than mere tools; they act as essential bridges to the subconscious. They bypass the analytical, sceptical often judgemental mind by slipping effortlessly into the deeper parts of the mind where transformation is waiting to occur. However, to grasp their true power, we must first explore how they work. Why do they resonate? What makes them uniquely suited for healing and growth?

A metaphor is a window into how the mind structures our perception of reality. When a client says, "I feel like I'm drowning in work," they aren't just talking about their tasks; they're conveying the emotional weight of their experience. The subconscious mind doesn't communicate in straightforward terms; it uses imagery, sensations, and emotions to express itself.

In hypnotherapy, metaphors are utilised to engage with the subconscious's unique language. These are more than just means to grasp a client's viewpoint; they offer fresh perspectives; reframes that unlock new possibilities. Picture guiding the client who feels overwhelmed to envision themselves as a swimmer finding a buoy or learning to float. This story instils the notion that not only is survival achievable, but mastery is within reach.

If metaphors really are seeds, then stories act as the gentle wind that directs them from whence they come to their eventual resting place, in the fertile soil of the human mind. A well-crafted story may contain layers of meaning, resonating with the client's reality and various individual aspects of the client's experience.

The beauty of storytelling in hypnotherapy resides in its fluidity and flexibility. Some stories are universal yet can still resonate differently with each individual, such as the phoenix that rises from the ashes. Other stories can be profoundly personal, crafted to mirror the client's distinct path.

Consider a client struggling with self-worth. Imagine sharing a story about a tarnished silver serving spoon that has remained buried in the soil for many years. Overlooked by passersby until one day, someone picks it up, polishes it, and reveals its enduring beauty and the intricacy of its engraving. This story may resonate, not because it directly addresses the client's issue; rather because it speaks to the client's subconscious. Just like the silver spoon, it invites the client to get curious and look beyond the superficial to see the inherent beauty, individuality and value that can be found just below the surface.

Every therapeutic story, like that of the forgotten spoon, follows a defined path, whether it's implied or stated outright. In hypnotherapy, this structure frequently reflects the client's personal journey.

The beginning of a story can establish familiarity for the client, creating rapport and drawing the client further in. As the narrative introduces struggles or challenges that subtly echo the client's own difficulties the client connection deepens and pathways to transformation or moments of triumph are introduced, planting seeds of hope and possibility.

For example, a client burdened by anxiety may find comfort in a therapeutic story about someone wandering through a dense fog, uncertain of the path ahead. Unable to see where future choices lead, the fog can elicit a foreboding feeling of impending danger about the path ahead in all its uncertainty and unfamiliarity. For the client, the fog may symbolise anxiety; an all-encompassing, disorienting and ever-present force. As the story continues, the character may find as they move forward one step at a time, the fog begins to lighten, and the pathway forward slowly comes into view revealing further choices as the path ahead divides. Relying on inner wisdom the character intuitively knows the right path which seems somehow brighter. Each well considered step is leading the character out of the fog and into the clearing, where everything begins to become clear.

Even if our clients don't completely understand all the symbolism, they can start to absorb the message. Their curiosity and desire to explore the deeper meanings allow them to recognise their own inner wisdom and resources. This helps them transition from the unsettling feelings of impending danger to a state of calm and clarity as previous unpleasant feelings gradually begin to dissipate, just like the fog.

When we construct stories or metaphors for our clients in hypnotherapy, we must be acutely aware that best outcomes are generally not achieved through a one-size-fits-all script. The story must resonate with the client's specific needs, experiences, and importantly their choice of language. We must listen deeply to the client's narrative, language patterns and choice of words and reflect these back in a way that is both familiar and transformative. This is where the art of hypnotherapy shines.

For instance, a client who is passionate about gardening may relate more profoundly to a metaphor about a seed's transformation into a tree, by developing strong roots, firmly connecting it to the ground, combined with a narrative describing how it has weathered many storms by learning to bend and be flexible. On the other hand, a client with a passion for sailing might find meaning in a story about a ship braving a wild storm by dropping the masts, reducing resistance and motoring into the calm waters of a protected cove until the storm passes. By grounding metaphors in the client's experiences, you help them recall challenges they have already overcome and allow them to acknowledge their ability to see the bigger picture, build an expectancy for change and be active participants in their own therapeutic journey.

For those of you who are already seeing clients or who have had your own experiences with Hypnotherapy, we must be aware that not all clients readily embrace metaphors or stories. Many clients are highly analytical or even sceptical about the process of hypnotherapy and the efficacy of these strange stories. In such cases we need to respect the client's perspective, so as not to break rapport, we must always connect with them where they are at that moment. Instead of presenting contradictory information, which again may create resistance and threaten rapport in certain clients, we can frame our stories as invitations to get curious about other possibilities. Dissociation is a good technique to utilise here as the story is about someone else, as it is often easier to find solutions when we are on the outside looking in.

For analytical clients, we may say, "I'm reminded of something that might resonate with your situation..." or "a colleague of mine was recently in a very similar situation and they overcame these challenges by ….." Narratives such as this can subtly encourage the client to engage with the story on their own terms and find their own solutions.

It is also important to remember, if we consider metaphors to be like seeds, then it follows that they may not yield immediate or dramatic results. The subconscious will often process these thoughts, suggestions and metaphors at its own pace. It may be hours, days, weeks, or even months later that the client may recall the story and draw strength or insights from it. Even more subtle than that, things may just begin to change for no apparent reason.

I once had a woman comeback to me two months after a 'stop-smoking session' stating that one day she just woke up and no longer desired to smoke. It was abhorrent to her. She wanted to let me know and thank me, as she said she knew it was a seed that was sown in the session that had taken root and continued to grow.

This leads me to discuss the ripple effect of a good metaphor or story. In fact, we could say that the true power of metaphor and story in hypnotherapy lies in its ability to ripple out in positive, often far-reaching ways over time and across various contexts. A single metaphor, therefore, can spark a cascade of realisations, and inspire a lifetime of change.

I recall working with a client who described life as overwhelming. Her house was in disarray with cupboards overflowing in every room and she did not know where to begin. She felt so overwhelmed by the thought of the task ahead that she sat in inertia doing nothing at all.

We crafted a story of a woman I once knew in a similar situation who had a pending open for inspection of her home. There was so much to do she didn't think it was even possible, until she decided that she didn't need to take on the whole task all at once. Rather she decided to only clear and tidy one shelf at a time, and when she was finished with the shelves, she would do the draws. Over the period of many weeks, she had cleared all the shelves and all the draws, and her house was ready well before the open inspection.

After the session my client thought this was a strategy she could employ. She decided that she was going to do only one shelf each day, an achievable task. The next day she would clear another shelf, and so on, and day after day she would be making visible progress. An easy task we both agreed. I suggested that she should ignore the other rooms and other shelves only venturing into the room in question to enjoy how satisfied she was with the shelf that she had tidied. I also asked her to peruse her work and really congratulate herself on a job well done, at least three times a day, but she was definitely only to do one shelf a day.

Erickson called this prescribing the problem; by only allowing her to clear one shelf she was being subtly encouraged in a paradoxical way to consciously engage in the very behaviour she wanted to stop, that of inertia or procrastination. When this is done within a strategic and intentional framework of really appreciating her results and feeling how good it was to achieve completion of the task, she was able to break the cycle of inertia.

By the time of our next visit, seven days later when there should have been only seven shelves cleared and tidied, she was able to tell me she had already tidied two entire rooms including drawers and two large double cupboards containing many more shelves than the seven agreed. She was also well on her way to finishing the third bedroom.

Her newfound satisfaction and pride were visible. By making small, positive actions clearing one "shelf" at a time, and enjoying the pleasure of her results, she was able to 'see' the shelves as manageable steps that broke the pattern of inaction. Once she began to see progress and feel how good it felt, she said she couldn't help herself, she had to do more.

As hypnotherapists, we are, at our core, storytellers.

We gently hold space for our clients and the stories they bring, weaving in metaphors, imagery and story to guide them toward healing and growth. It is important that we don't rewrite their endings, rather we offer new possibilities, and fresh perspectives allowing them to imagine the next chapter differently. Sometimes this is through a quiet metaphor or a story that surreptitiously slips beneath the surface and stirs something deep.

Next time you sit with your client, I encourage you to really listen, not just to the words, but to the meaning beneath the words. Notice the metaphors they already use, the language of their inner world. What images or symbols are they using that speak louder than words? Look for the opportunity to offer them a new image, a new story or metaphor that gently opens the doorway to glimpse the possibility of hope as it invites them to take the next creative step forward on their path to healing.

Chapter Twelve

HYPNOTHERAPY IN HARMONY WITH OTHER THERAPIES

Dave Elman used to say *"Hypnosis is not a panacea, nor is it a replacement for medical or psychological treatment. It is, however, a powerful adjunct, one that can help unlock the resources of the mind to support healing, growth, and change."*

Many variations of this sentiment appear throughout Elman's work, especially in the book "Hypnotherapy" (1964) one of the first books on hypnotherapy that I read, and one that truly influenced my hypnotherapeutic direction.

Therefore, as we explore the integration of hypnotherapy with other diverse therapeutic modalities, it's crucial to remember that, as hypnotherapists, we operate within an ethical framework, engaging only in areas where we have received appropriate training. Thus, we proceed on this journey with care and with the understanding that each therapeutic modality possesses its own theoretical foundations, methodologies, and ethical considerations.

It is the responsibility of all practitioners to recognise their limitations and adhere to these professional boundaries. While blending different approaches can certainly foster a dynamic synergy, doing so without adequate training and comprehension may result in confusion or inconsistency for clients.

I think it is very safe to say that in the ever-evolving field of wellness and mental health, no single approach holds all the answers. This raises a crucial question: How can we effectively blend different therapeutic modalities to enhance healing?

Just as a symphony blends the sounds of multiple instruments to create a harmonious masterpiece, combining therapies can yield powerful results, addressing the complex layers of the human experience. Hypnotherapy, with its unique ability to access the deeper subconscious mind, is particularly well-suited to integrate with other therapies. This integration is not just beneficial; it can be transformative, enhancing the impact of each modality and facilitating deeper, more holistic healing.

Hypnotherapy and Cognitive-Behavioural Therapy

Cognitive-behavioural therapy (CBT) is amongst the most prevalent and research-backed methods in mental health treatment. So, what contributes to CBT's effectiveness? Its emphasis on recognising and transforming negative thought processes complement the goals of hypnotherapy exceptionally well. While CBT predominantly functions within the conscious mind, hypnotherapy can explore the deeper layers of the mind, targeting the subconscious beliefs and emotional injuries that often underlie these thought patterns.

Imagine an individual dealing with social anxiety, with CBT they can begin to confront their fear of rejection by reshaping negative thoughts and adopting new behaviours. However, if a lingering childhood memory of humiliation is left unaddressed, their advancement may plateau. Hypnotherapy can assist in revealing and reframing that memory, helping the person to let go of its emotional charge. When combined, these two therapeutic approaches can present an holistic strategy, tackling both the conscious symptoms and the underlying causes of anxiety.

In practice, blending CBT and hypnotherapy can be seamless. A therapist might start a session with CBT techniques to explore a client's conscious thoughts and then transition into hypnosis to reinforce positive changes at the subconscious level. Alternatively, a hypnotherapy session could be followed by CBT-based homework, empowering the client to be aware of problematic thoughts or patterns and implement their new strategies into daily life. All successes are subsequently introduced into the ongoing hypnotherapy sessions reinforcing the client's progress. By combining these modalities, clients achieve a richer therapeutic experience that equips them with the tools they need to thrive.

Hypnotherapy and Mindfulness-Based Practices

How do we invite more awareness and presence into our therapeutic work? Both mindfulness and hypnotherapy offer pathways to reflect and explore our internal environment. Both aim to deepen our connection to thoughts, emotions, and our internal narrative that exists within the stories we tell ourselves and others. Utilising mindfulness and hypnotherapy together can significantly enhance therapeutic outcomes by integrating their unique strengths.

Mindfulness gently teaches us to witness our inner experiences with curiosity and compassion, establishing a solid foundation for heightened awareness. It allows individuals to maintain an observational vantage point from which to explore their memories and emotions, promoting a non-judgmental understanding of unresolved issues or limiting beliefs. This practice also enables the observation of negative thought patterns without attachment. Hypnotherapy complements mindfulness by opening the door to transformation, guiding the mind to explore, reframe, and release old patterns while stepping into new ways of thinking, feeling, and being. The skilful combination of mindfulness and hypnotherapy creates a potent synergy for personal transformation, strengthening the likelihood of successfully integrating more helpful thoughts, feelings, and emotions at a subconscious level.

This heightened self-awareness is beneficial before entering hypnotherapy, as it allows clients to identify specific issues or patterns they wish to address. Engaging in mindfulness techniques can help clients relax and focus, making it easier for them to enter a hypnotic state. Mindful practices can easily be incorporated within a hypnotic induction to direct our clients to notice subtle changes in their body and mind as they progress deeper into the hypnotic state.

Mindful preparation may reduce anxiety, increasing receptivity to suggestions made during the hypnotherapy session. Once mindful awareness is cultivated in our clients, hypnotherapy can take it further, enabling the exploration and correction of subconscious patterns that are currently inhibiting their health and happiness. When skilfully combined, these two methodologies not only improve self-awareness but can also enable deep transformations at the very core of one's being.

Mindfulness tools combined with hypnotic practices can also be utilised when tasking our clients to do the out of session work that will enhance their outcomes, such as thought awareness and self-hypnotic practices, and tools to regulate their emotions, making it easier to process challenging experiences.

The combination of both modalities can lead to long-lasting changes by reinforcing new insights and behaviours. Mindfulness outside the therapeutic sessions fosters ongoing self-reflection and awareness, allowing clients to recognise and maintain the progress achieved during hypnotherapy sessions. In essence, the integration of mindfulness and hypnotherapy provides a holistic framework that addresses both conscious and subconscious aspects of the mind, empowering individuals to achieve deeper insights, emotional healing, and sustained personal growth.

For instance, someone battling chronic stress will most probably struggle to quieten their racing mind. When we introduce mindfulness techniques, we demonstrate to our clients how they can recognise their thoughts, detach from those that are not helpful such as anxious thoughts, limiting thoughts or ruminations, and in doing so they cultivate a feeling of calm and self-empowerment as they begin to recognise the things that they can control. Hypnotherapy can then build on this foundation, helping the individual to neurologically rewire their previous automatic subconscious responses to stress. By combining mindfulness with hypnotherapy, individuals not only observe their thoughts but can play an active role in reshaping them.

Most of you will now understand that you are already utilising mindfulness in your client sessions, as it is a natural part of the hypnotic process. Hypnotherapy naturally and effectively combines practices that incorporate mindful language such as focusing on the breath and observing bodily sensations, all designed to deepen the trance state and the client's connection to the present moment. This narrowed focus of attention supports integration of new ideas and empowers our clients to change their state whenever and wherever they need to.

Hypnotherapy and Somatic Therapies

In the words of Bessel van der Kolk "The Body Keeps the Score,". In fact, in 2014 he first published a book by that name that has since gained significant popularity and has sold over one million copies worldwide.

His book explores the profound impact of trauma on both the mind and body. Van der Kolk, who is a leading expert in the field of trauma, emphasises that traumatic experiences can and do lead to physical and emotional symptoms, affecting an individual's overall well-being. He discusses in the book how trauma can lead to various physical ailments and illuminates the intimate connection between emotional experiences and bodily sensations.

Van der Kolk advocates for the use of an holistic approach including somatic therapies, mindfulness, and body-based approaches to help individuals process and heal from trauma. He emphasises that effective treatment must address both mind and body.

So, what occurs when we recognise the relationship between the mind and body?

The mind and body are so closely intertwined that emotional experiences can often manifest as physical sensations or symptoms within the body. Somatic therapies, which emphasise the release of trauma and tension from the body can serve as a natural complement to Hypnotherapy's exploration of the subconscious mind.

There are many physical manifestations emanating from emotional experiences. Many common ones that can be observed in the hypnotherapy clinic may present as tension and tightness, originating from stress or anxiety, particularly in the neck, shoulders, or jaw. Pain may present after emotional distress, due to chronic activation of the sympathetic nervous system, contributing to chronic pain conditions, headaches or back pain. Changes to the cardiovascular system in the form of elevated heart rate, elevated blood pressure or cardiac arrhythmias such as tachycardia or palpitations are not uncommon in times of extreme stress or trauma. This often combined with changes in breathing patterns such as rapid or shallow breathing can lead to ongoing feelings of anxiety.

Digestive Issues are also common due to the effect of stress on the gastrointestinal system, leading to stomach aches, nausea, or changes in appetite or even gastric ulcers. Fatigue is often the result from prolonged emotional stress and can result in physical exhaustion and reduced energy levels. The skin can also be affected when emotions trigger skin conditions such as rashes or hives, and chronic stress can also weaken the immune system, making the body more susceptible to illness.

As you can begin to clearly see, every organ and every system in the body is impacted by stress and trauma. As the massive elephant in the room, sometimes overlooked by cognitive therapies alone, it becomes imperative to address this in our hypnotherapeutic sessions.

There are many ways to do this in a hypnotherapy session, some of which I will discuss briefly. First and foremost, when dealing with trauma, it is essential to establish safety for the client. We can do this by giving informed consent and detailed education about the process, creating clear boundaries and establishing an exit plan should the client need one, be it; a safe place or just letting them know they can open their eyes and exit the trance state at will.

In such situations, after establishing a 'safe place', I use a gentle induction method such as a mindful progressive muscle relaxation, with a breath focus, to guide the client into a comfortable state.

Clients are directed to notice different sensations in their body fostering a deeper connection to their physical self. They are instructed to notice if these areas have a feeling such as tightness, or heaviness, or perhaps if our client is more visual, the symptom may be represented by a colour. If there are areas of tension or discomfort that are connected to their emotions or experiences, they are asked to observe without judgment. Visualisation is utilised here to introduce healing, calming, cooling or warmth, whatever is required by the client. Heavy feelings are lightened, large areas are made smaller, intense colours are faded or changed and calming, healing imagery is introduced. The client is encouraged to explore what feels, looks or sound right for them as they imagine the release of tension or trauma from their body often using their breath or light as a tool for healing. Again, it is important for our clients to do what is meaningful to them as this is never a one-size-fits-all technique.

The client is directed to remain aware of the change in any physical sensations as they receive suggestions. In this way emotional changes can be integrated at a somatic level.

Positive solution focused suggestions based on connecting to resources, releasing the past, healing and empowerment to create change are given to reinforce the connection between their emotional and physical well-being.

Hypnotherapy can enhance body awareness, guiding clients to tune into areas of calm, comfort and clarity, therefore upon reorientation clients are encouraged to notice these changes in bodily sensations. We then give our clients the space to discuss their experiences and insights and to carry these with them after the session and into their day.

For example, you may imagine a hypnotherapist leading a client who has presented with anxiety related symptoms such as a tight chest, a clenched jaw or a ruminating mind to imagine sending a colour that represents relaxation, calm or clarity to the effected regions through hypnotic visualisation. At the same time suggestions of release, softening, fading, shrinking and peace can be strategically given in time with the clients longer slower exhalation, combined with affirmation of the great work the client is doing each time a muscle release is observed. This hypnotic approach supports physical relaxation and transformation of the specific symptoms while reinforcing the client's ability to direct the mind-body responses by activating the parasympathetic nervous system leading to holistic healing.

When we, as therapists, integrate hypnotherapy and somatic practices we can amplify the beneficial effects of therapy by accessing a relaxed, safe state where clients feel comfortable to explore and release emotional and physical tension. Incorporating somatic work into hypnotherapeutic sessions can deepen the healing process and provide clients with valuable tools for managing their emotional and physical well-being far beyond the hypnotherapy room.

Hypnotherapy and Creative Therapies

Creativity is a natural expression of the subconscious mind and the hypnotic trance state, one that has no need of logic or reality, the perfect playground therefore for creative healing. Typically woven into most hypnotherapy sessions, creativity acts as the vessel that guides us through the fantasy and enchantment of the deepest chambers, monoliths, and labyrinths of the subconscious mind. The work we accomplish in this space can be as transformative as a caterpillar discovering its wings as it emerges from the chrysalis to soar freely as a beautiful butterfly.

Creative therapy comes in many forms, directed hypnotic suggestion as previously discussed, but also through art, music, or drama, which can be perfect pairings with hypnotherapy. In fact, I would postulate that most epic creative inspiration arises from a trance-like flow state, where art and music combine with the powerful subconscious potential to soar high above the everyday 'ordinary'.

Art and music can effectively assist in tapping into the emotions and memories that often words alone struggle to reach, providing a powerful outlet for healing and self-discovery.

For example, a client working through grief might find it difficult to articulate their feelings in traditional therapy. Guided by a hypnotherapist, they could enter a relaxed state where they visualise their emotions as colours or shapes. This is particularly effective when working with children. The client may then imagine translating these images into a painting or drawing that reinterprets the original meaning to one that is more healing. This process may be done in the privacy and creativity of the client's own mind, or an actual drawing may be created, often after the session as a homework task, to allow for further emotional release and processing as the client gains deeper insights into their inner world and its representations.

Similarly, music therapy and hypnotherapy can complement one another beautifully. Music has a remarkable ability to access and evoke memories due to its profound connection to our emotions and experiences creating the ideal environment for hypnosis. Have you ever heard a piece of music and been immediately transported back to a past experience when you heard the music played? Generally, there will be an emotional charge to these memories. Perhaps it was a moving piece of music played at a funeral, or a song played at a party when you had your first kiss. Either way the music has the uncanny ability to take you right back there in an instant. Now picture a session where soothing music plays softly as the therapist guides the client through visualisations and suggestion to enhance the therapeutic impact of both modalities.

Studies show that music activates various brain regions involved in memory processing, including the hippocampus and amygdala. This neurological engagement enhances the retrieval of stored, often emotionally significant memories allowing them to be accessed and processed safely within the hypnotic state.

Another way to incorporate music into a hypnotic session is by utilisation. Music lyrics from a client's favourite song can also be utilised to inspire and uplift the client when presented as part of a well-formed therapeutic suggestion. People also often create personal narratives around specific songs, weaving the themes into their life stories. This too can be useful as specific inspirational themes, words or phrases can be used whilst in trance to connect the client to these narratives, thus strengthening emotional and cognitive connections to their resources.

Hypnotherapy and Energy Healing

There are many energy healing modalities, such as Reiki, Acupuncture or chakra balancing that concentrate on restoring the body's natural energy flow. These practices align seamlessly with hypnotherapy's focus on establishing harmony between the conscious and subconscious mind, creating a powerful synergy for holistic healing.

During a hypnotherapy session, the therapist may encourage the client to visualise energy flowing freely throughout their body, helping to release blocks or tension. This imagery enhances energy healing techniques, amplifying their impact and fostering a deeper sense of balance and well-being.

For example, a client suffering from chronic fatigue could benefit from the combined approaches of hypnotherapy and energy healing. While the hypnotherapist delves into subconscious beliefs regarding overwork or lack of self-worth, focus can also be directed towards restoring, replenishing and revitalising the body's energy. This integrated treatment plan effectively addresses both the mental and physical aspects of the presenting issues.

THE FUTURE OF INTEGRATED THERAPIES

"Trauma is not just an event that took place sometime in the past; it is also the imprint left by that experience on mind, brain, and body." (van der Kolk, 2014), *The Body Keeps the Score*.

As the landscape of healing continues to evolve, we are privy to witnessing a quiet but profound shift in how therapeutic modalities relate to one another. The once rigid lines that separated different approaches are becoming more fluid, dissolving in response to both lived clinical experience and the growing body of empirical evidence and research that underscores the interconnection of mind, body, and spirit.

This shift we are witnessing is not solely philosophical. it is deeply rooted in emerging evidence from neuroscience, somatic psychology, and integrative medicine, which together reveal the complex interplay between internal states and the body's capacity to heal. (van der Kolk, 2014).

Alongside these developments, technology is also playing its part in shaping the future of care. It is enabling practitioners to offer more personalised, flexible, and hybrid experiences, blending modalities in ways that were previously unforeseen such as telehealth, app-supported self-hypnosis, and integrative group work that draws on both live and digital modalities. These innovations reflect a broader cultural movement toward accessibility and self-agency in the healing process.

At the heart of this integration is the central principle: healing is most effective when it is holistic. Hypnotherapy has a particularly important role to play here. Its unique capacity to access the subconscious mind, the home of stored emotions, symbolic imagery, and internalised beliefs, make it a natural complement to many other modalities. Whether paired with somatic therapies, energy work, trauma-informed counselling, or even medical treatment, hypnotherapy can act as a gentle but powerful catalyst to healing.

In this way, hypnotherapy becomes more than a standalone practice, it becomes a bridge that can link talk-based therapeutic exploration with embodied awareness, or spiritual insight with psychological clarity. It allows the client's inner experience to be met and engaged with on multiple levels, facilitating a shift not just in symptoms, but in meaning, narrative, and somatic expression.

Chapter Thirteen

SAFELY EXPLORING THE PAST TO HEAL THE PRESENT – REGRESSION IN HYPNOTHERAPY

"Progress isn't always achieved through forward motion. Sometimes the truest path ahead is achieved by going in the opposite direction."
Danielle Aitken

A word of Caution, the critical word in this chapter title is safely. When we seek to heal the past, we must tread carefully to avoid unintentionally re-traumatising our clients. Regression therapy is a powerful and insightful tool, yet it necessitates a thoughtful and deliberate approach. Practitioners must be acutely aware that exploring memories long buried can sometimes unearth deep emotions and unresolved trauma.

Regression therapy is based on the idea that our subconscious mind holds memories, emotions, and beliefs from past experiences which are often outside of our conscious awareness. These unresolved memories can present themselves as anxiety, phobias, self-doubt, or detrimental behavioural patterns.

Our current challenges frequently stem from unresolved experiences in our past. Regression in hypnotherapy serves as a powerful tool, enabling clients to revisit these significant moments, not to relive the associated pain, but rather to reframe and release it. This chapter delves into the mechanics of regression, its effectiveness, and the profound transformations it can facilitate.

As we know, when in hypnosis, clients enter an altered brain state. This altered state allows access to the subconscious mind and enables the processing of memories from the past to be facilitated in a way than is often not achieved by the conscious mind. When practiced effectively during hypnosis, regression can be utilised to enable clients to safely recall, review and reprocess events that may have contributed to their current difficulties. Dr. Brian Weiss, a pioneer in the field of regression therapy, notes that accessing the subconscious helps clients to release emotional blockages and fosters a deeper understanding of themselves (Weiss, 1988).

I often hear therapists and even tutors assert that regression should not be employed in therapy. This claim baffles me, as I cannot envision hypnotherapy without it. I have conveyed to my students and supervisees that even the simplest and most commonly practiced search for past resources, such as reflecting on last week to identify changes, recalling a joyful moment, revisiting a favourite place or activity, or accessing feelings of empowerment, constitutes a form of regression. Whenever we encourage our clients to think back beyond the present moment, whether it's just moments before they entered the room perhaps with apprehension today or to remember yesterday's sunset, last week's disagreement, last year's birthday celebration, or events from long ago, we are utilising regression.

Reflecting on my many years of practice, I am especially struck by those clients who have left a lasting impression due to the transformative outcomes they have achieved. When I consider these clients, it is regression therapy that stands out in my mind as the profoundly effective treatment that finally helped them reach their goals. These are the clients who often have tried everything and consulted numerous specialists prior to arriving at the hypnotherapy clinic, from general practitioners and paediatricians to psychologists, anaesthetists, pain management teams, and even psychiatrists. These are individuals who have endured a myriad of hardships over many years but have not yet given up, often turning to hypnotherapy as their last resort. The very same clients who subsequently achieved spectacular results, remarkably finding relief after just a few short hypnotherapy sessions.

This successful group have made a significant mark on my own journey as a practitioner. They are the standout clients, the ones I will never forget, and I am grateful for the ability to have utilised regression therapy in such a way that has allowed me to have been part of their collective journeys.

Having said that, it is essential to remember, if a client indicates that they do not wish to explore the past, then regression is not the appropriate therapy to employ, no matter how much the therapist believes it would be helpful. It is essential that we always respect the needs and wishes of our clients if we do not wish to re-traumatise them. Our clients are the authorities on their own experiences, and this should be recognised and honoured.

So how do we responsibly utilise regression, to ensure the safety and well-being of clients? Firstly, it is essential that therapists only utilise techniques for which they are properly trained, competent, and confident. Each therapeutic method carries its own unique challenges and requires a deep understanding of the underlying principles. Therefore, not only are therapists required to work solely with techniques and principles for which they are fully trained, they must also engage in essential continuous professional development, as required by all reputable associations, in order to stay informed and skilled in the techniques they employ.

Before embarking on a regression journey, it is vital for hypnotherapists to establish a safe and supportive environment. Clients are encouraged to communicate their concerns and any apprehensions, making sure they grasp the regression process and what it might be like to revisit delicate experiences. By promoting a respectful and cooperative environment, therapists can assist clients in managing the difficult emotions that may surface during the session.

Once a hypnotic state is reached, the conscious mind steps aside, allowing the subconscious to take centre stage. The therapist uses gentle prompts and non-leading language, such as, "Imagine tracing that troublesome feeling back to the very first time you experienced it," to guide the client to a specific moment in time for exploration. Before proceeding, it is crucial to ask, "Is this the first time you ever experienced that feeling?" If the answer is yes, you continue; if no, guidance is provided to take the client even further back to just before the initial incident, often referred to as the initiating event. This step is essential, as failing to reach the initiating event increases the likelihood that symptoms of the presenting issue will remain unresolved.

The initiating event often uncovers the origin of the issue, such as a childhood event, an emotional wound, or a limiting belief. Once at the initiating event, if the client revisits an experience from when they were seven years old, they are encouraged to imagine themselves at that age now and explore the situation through the eyes their seven-year-old self, speaking in the present tense, however this must only be done when the client feels safe to do so. If the client does not feel safe, dissociation techniques may be employed.

The client is encouraged to become curious as they explore the circumstances, thoughts, feelings, emotions and beliefs surrounding the event. All of these insights are noted down by the therapist. Once fully explored the therapist helps the client reframe their perspective by bringing in the adult self and exploring what their older wiser self knows now that they didn't know when they were a young child with limited resources. For example, a child who felt unworthy after being criticised by a parent can, as an adult, recognise that the criticism reflected the struggles and short comings of the parent and had little to do with them. They can view themselves as just a normal little child doing normal childlike things.

During regression therapists need to remain vigilant for signs of distress, checking in with the client to see if they are happy to sit with any disturbing emotions that may arise. Clients are gently supported through this process as they uncover the insights arising from the events that have stimulated present day issues and use their current resources to reframe them into something they can now deal with.

Utilising a mindful and informed approach, regression therapy can lead to transformative outcomes for our clients as they get to explore the past from a safe vantage point with confidence and access to their resources, emerging with new insights that allow for healing to occur.

The session concludes by deepening the trance and offering any client insights back to the client as hypnotic suggestions designed to reinforce positive revelations, beliefs and emotions, that have been discovered during the session, allowing the client to move forward with clarity toward healing.

CASE STUDY: SAM'S FEAR OF PUBLIC SPEAKING

Sam, a 42-year-old well respected manager of a well-known national company, came to therapy with a crippling fear of public speaking. Despite being highly knowledgeable in his field, he avoided presentations, networking events, and media appearances, which impacted his career growth.

The Regression Session:

During hypnosis, Sam was guided to the initiating event of his fear. He recalled a vivid memory of starting a new school when he was six years old. Sitting in class on his first day of school as the new boy, during a class spelling bee. His turn came around and all the three letter words that he knew, bat, cat, dog, mat had been spelled. Sam had to admit to his new class that he didn't know any other words. He felt stupid and not as good as the others in his class. The teacher made a dismissive comment, and the class laughed. In that moment, Sam internalised the beliefs, 'I am a bad speller', 'everyone knows I'm not as smart as the other kids', He believed that he wasn't good enough and people would laugh at him.

Sam was then able to observe the memory from a dissociated adult perspective. He recognised that his teacher's comment was inappropriate and didn't define his abilities. He was able to replace the belief of I am not good enough, with a more empowering one: 'I was just a little boy in a strange new environment, and I didn't get the support I deserved'. 'I am knowledgeable, capable, and confident'.

After the session Sam was asked to reflect on what he learned from the session, and to remember the insights from the session regarding the things he didn't know when he was six, but that he does know now. He reported significant improvements. He began speaking at smaller events, gradually building confidence. Six months later, he gave a keynote presentation at a professional conference whilst confidently writing on a white board in front of a large audience, a milestone he never thought possible.

Some of the most profound outcomes of regression therapy, when conducted skilfully by well-trained practitioners, arise from the client's capacity to safely access and heal unresolved emotional wounds that have been subconsciously influencing their present experience, often without conscious awareness.

This process can therefore help clients break free from entrenched patterns and habits rooted in the past. By reframing these experiences using present-day insights and internal resources, the emotional charge associated with them can be significantly altered. As a result, clients frequently experience a deepened sense of self-understanding and emotional liberation.

However, it is essential to once again state clearly that hypnotic regression must always be approached with care. Practitioners must take great caution to avoid the use of leading questions that could inadvertently contribute to the formation of false memories. The therapist's primary focus must remain on the client's well-being at all times.

Clients should be well informed that memories accessed under hypnosis are not necessarily literal or factually accurate. This is due to the nature of the subconscious mind, which processes experiences through a complex system of filtering, distorting, and generalising. In this way, memory is not a perfect recording but a reconstruction, often influenced by emotional states and imaginative processes. As such, the therapeutic goal is not factual verification but rather emotional resolution and integration.

Bearing this in mind let's explore how much information we do process at any given moment. the overall rate at which we consciously process information is surprisingly slow, about 10 bits per second. This is the equivalent of making one or two clear choices or reading two short words per second or understanding a few simple sensory details like recognising a colour, a sound or a word's meaning. In comparison, our sensory systems, such as vision, hearing, and touch, collect information from the surroundings at an astonishing rate of about 1 billion bits per second. (Sauerbrei & Pruszynski, 2025). This indicates that the brain is significantly filtering and condensing a massive amount of sensory data into a small stream of information that is readily available for conscious thought. Given this, it is not surprising that our memory recall cannot be depended upon to be absolutely accurate. This prompts an important question, how does the brain prioritise, process, and make decisions about what information to filter into that small stream that becomes available for conscious thought?

The rest of this huge amount of information is handled automatically by the subconscious mind, which filters out what it considers unimportant or expected. More than this, recent research indicates that the brain doesn't just react to the world around us, it predicts what will happen and filters information based on those predictions (Kilner, Friston, & Frith, 2007).

Interesting, isn't it? Those heated arguments with family over the years, where you're absolutely certain something happened one way, while a relative insists, just as strongly, that the complete opposite is true. Even more baffling is when sometimes, a person has heard a story repeated so often that they end up writing themselves into it, despite not even having been there at the time. In psychology they called this process confabulation. This is when a person unintentionally fabricates or distorts a memory filling in the gaps with their own version of the story that they believe to be true.

This filtering system helps us stay focused, but it also means we're only ever seeing a narrow slice of reality. Models such as the **Global Workspace Theory** describe consciousness as a spotlight: it illuminates one thing at a time, while everything else remains in the dark.

And for all the multitaskers out there, I'm sorry to say it, but the brain doesn't truly multitask. It simply switches rapidly from one point of focus to another, which is far less efficient than we like to believe.

When we pull together all the 'bits of information' presented so far, a clearer picture begins to emerge; our reality and our memories are not fixed recordings but constructed experiences that are shaped by the small fragments of information we happen to focus on. In hypnotherapy, there's a saying: *what we focus on, we strengthen*, and this may be why.

Regression in hypnotherapy, therefore, is ultimately a journey of self-discovery. An opportunity for clients to shine a light in the space between past-experience and present perception. By working with the subconscious mind, regression therapy allows us to gently update the internal filters that have shaped our present experience.

Although we cannot change the past, and may not even recall it with accuracy, we can change how we interpret, respond to, and hold the experiences we remember. Through this process of insight and integration, old emotional wounds can be healed, and the future no longer needs to be shaped by the shadows of the past.

As Carl Jung so aptly put it: *"Until you make the unconscious conscious, it will direct your life, and you will call it fate."*

Chapter Fourteen

RECLAIMING THE LIGHT: HYPNOTHERAPY FOR DEPRESSION

This chapter highlights the transformative potential of hypnotherapy for depression, weaving together neuroscience, therapeutic techniques, and Sally's inspiring case study.

Depression is like a silent adversary casting its shadow over every aspect of life as it quietly undermines its unfortunate recipient. It can dull life's vibrant colours, stifle joy, silence optimism, and isolate the sufferer in a relentless heavy fog of hopelessness. Yet, beneath its heavy weight lies a truth often forgotten: the mind and body when working together in harmony possess a profound capacity for healing.

Hypnotherapy offers a gentle yet effective way to lift the fog of depression by working directly with the subconscious mind. It helps uncover underlying causes, shift unhelpful beliefs, and importantly, build an expectation of change, rekindling a sense of hope. Where depression lives, hope does not. Many clients who are experiencing depression express feeling hopeless, therefore creating hope is an essential process in our clients rediscovering the path toward healing.

This chapter explores the interplay between depression and the subconscious mind, the neuroscience underpinning hypnotherapy's effectiveness, and the transformative potential of this therapeutic modality.

To discuss this topic, we must firstly understand depression and again I reiterate, we as hypnotherapists, must only work within our areas of training and competency. Also, as hypnotherapists, we never advise our clients to cease or reduce any medications. Any such actions must always be undertaken in consultation between the client and their treating physician.

Depression is more than a temporary state of sadness or a response to challenging life events. It is a complex and persistent condition that can deeply affect a person's emotions, thoughts, and behaviours. Common symptoms include enduring feelings of sadness or emotional numbness, a loss of interest or pleasure in previously enjoyed activities, low energy or fatigue, difficulty concentrating, sleep disturbances such as insomnia or hypersomnia, and pervasive feelings of worthlessness or guilt (American Psychiatric Association)

While the causes of depression are multifactorial, encompassing genetic vulnerabilities, neurobiological imbalances, psychosocial stressors, and environmental influences, the influence of subconscious processes is often overlooked. Subconscious patterns, shaped by early experiences and internalised beliefs, can silently reinforce cycles of hopelessness, self-doubt, and emotional pain.

Clinical hypnotherapy, which facilitates access to these underlying patterns through focused attention and therapeutic suggestion, offers a pathway to identify and reframe self-limiting beliefs that may be contributing to depressive states (Alladin, 2016). Uncovering and working with these deeper layers may be key to lasting change and recovery.

Recent neuroscience research has helped us understand more about how depression affects the brain. It shows that depression isn't just a response to difficult circumstances, it also involves changes in how certain parts of the brain function. According to Akil and Nestler (2023), the neurobiology of stress plays a significant role in vulnerability and resilience in major depression. These changes help explain why people with depression often feel stuck, overwhelmed, or unable to shift their thinking.

One key area affected is the prefrontal cortex, which plays a major role in regulating emotions and solving problems. In people with depression, this area tends to be under-active, making it harder to manage emotions and cope with challenges.

At the same time, the amygdala, the part of the brain involved in emotional responses, often becomes overactive. This can lead to heightened sensitivity to negative emotions, reinforcing cycles of worry, sadness, or hopelessness.

Another system that's affected is the default mode network (DMN), which is linked to self-reflection and internal thoughts. When this network is overly active, it can lead to excessive rumination, constantly thinking about the past or judging oneself harshly.

Finally, the stress response system, known as the HPA axis, can also become overworked. Ongoing stress may keep this system on high alert, leading to higher levels of the stress hormone cortisol, which has been linked to increased symptoms of depression.

Clinical hypnotherapy can play a supportive role in addressing these brain-based patterns. By promoting deep relaxation and calming the stress response, hypnotherapy helps quiet the mind and reduce emotional reactivity. It also supports the brain's natural ability to rewire itself. Neuroplasticity therefore makes it easier to shift unhelpful thinking and create space for new, more empowering beliefs. (Alladin, 2016)

Hypnotherapy is uniquely positioned to help clients facing depression because it works directly with the subconscious mind, the storehouse of emotions, memories, and beliefs and automatic habits and patterns. It therefore has the capacity to get to the heart of what keeps individuals trapped in their pain and despair. It allows clients to explore the underlying emotional wounds or traumas contributing to their depression. This exploration can reveal insights, often not available to the conscious mind, that begin to open pathways for healing.

Through suggestion and guided imagery, clients may then begin the process of replacing limiting beliefs with empowering ones. For instance, transforming "I am useless" into "I am good enough" or "I am deserving of love and kindness" is a crucial step toward healing.

Hypnosis also promotes emotional regulation by activating the parasympathetic nervous system, creating a state of calm and reducing the overactivity of the amygdala. This tranquillity enables clearer, more rational thinking, paving the way for healthier emotional responses. The client may not have experienced this level of tranquillity in a long time, and thus the state of hypnosis in and of itself may act as a convincer to the client that change is possible. Clients often leave sessions feeling more connected to their inner strength as they begin to see that a brighter future, is not only possible, but is within reach.

Given the multifaceted nature of depression, certain therapeutic techniques have shown particular effectiveness in supporting clients through their emotional healing. Each method serves a distinct purpose, helping individuals navigate their internal landscape with greater clarity and ease.

One such technique is progressive muscle relaxation (PMR), which involves systematically relaxing muscle groups to induce a state of deep physical and mental calm. This practice has been shown to reduce physiological symptoms of stress by down-regulating activity in the amygdala and the hypothalamic-pituitary-adrenal (HPA) axis, both of which are often over-activated in individuals experiencing depression. By gently easing the body into a relaxed state, clients are better able to engage with their emotional experiences in a way that feels safe and grounded.

In this receptive state, tailored hypnotic suggestions can be introduced to support cognitive and emotional reframing. Rather than reinforcing self-defeating narratives or fixating on perceived failures, clients are guided to recognise their inner strengths and resources. This intentional redirection of attention can interrupt patterns of negative rumination and promote more adaptive ways of thinking (Alladin, 2016).

Regression Therapy can also be helpful as clients can be assisted to safely explore past experiences and uncover and heal from unresolved emotional wounds. This can be especially important for those whose depression has roots in childhood experiences or traumatic events. However, again with the words of Milton Erickson ringing in our ears, the future is of great importance for our depressed clients. The ability to future pace them into a life that is better, helps foster an expectation that life *can* be better. Our client's ability to visualise a hopeful future gives birth to motivation and a sense of purpose. This technique plants seeds of possibility and challenges the limiting beliefs that have kept them stagnant.

Likewise, Dr. Michael Yapko, prominent clinical psychologist and expert in the field of hypnotherapy and depression, emphasises the crucial role of building expectancy and hope into the therapeutic process. It is by harnessing the power of hypnotherapy that practitioners can facilitate a shift in the depressed clients' mindset, encouraging them to envision positive outcomes and new possibilities for their future.

Metaphors and stories can also be effectively utilised for our depressed clients, to bypass resistance and communicate directly with the subconscious mind. These symbolic narratives can resonate deeply, allowing clients to explore emotional truths in a gentle and indirect way.

For example, a depressed client might be guided to imagine nurturing a small seed and watching it grow into a strong, thriving tree, symbolising their own process of healing and development. Alternatively, they may be invited to recall a grand old tree on the foreshore that has weathered countless storms yet still stands tall and resilient, reflecting their inner strength and capacity to endure life's challenges. Such imagery can evoke hope, connection, and a sense of meaning, reinforcing the client's journey toward renewal.

CASE STUDY: SALLY'S JOURNEY

Background Sally, a 38-year-old nurse, sought hypnotherapy after struggling with depression for two years. The loss of her mother, who she had always had a distant relationship with, coupled with the stress of her demanding career, had left her feeling emotionally depleted. She described her days as "grey and heavy," filled with self-doubt and a persistent sense of imposter-syndrome and failure.

Sally had tried medication and talk therapy but found them insufficient in addressing her deep-rooted hopelessness. She arrived at her first session with a mix of scepticism and desperation, saying, "I've tried everything else. I don't know if this will work, but I'm willing to give it a go."

The pre-hypnotherapy work involved discussing with Sally the cognitive awareness tools that I would ask her to practice between sessions. She was asked to monitor her thoughts that were not helpful and redirect her focus to something more goal oriented, such as something she was grateful for. For Sally, this was her children. Importantly at this stage we developed a sense of what the future Sally would be like, feel like and how that version of herself would be living life. This was something that I asked Sally to focus on every day as we began the process of building the expectancy that life could be different and that change was possible. Importantly, these homework task are pivotal in creating changes in the neurology that has been running the depression rumination cycle.

The initial hypnotherapy session focused on building rapport and creating a safe space for Sally. Through progressive relaxation, she entered a light trance and experienced her first glimpse of inner calm. I introduced a metaphor, inviting her to imagine setting down the heavy backpack she had carried for years, symbolising her emotional burdens.

As she visualised this release, tears streamed down her face. For the first time in months, she felt a little lighter, a small, yet significant change.

During the second session we used regression therapy to explore the origins of Sally's depression by getting her to focus on the feelings that had brought her to therapy and tracking them back through time to observe where they began. She recalled a vivid childhood memory of her mother getting angry at her for bringing home a failed maths test result. After getting angry her mother stated you should be more like your sister. In that moment, Sally internalised the belief that she wasn't ever quite good enough.

We reframed this belief in trance as Sally was encouraged to use her current knowledge as a nurse and a mother to recognise what she now knows. She was able to confidently state that her mother's words were based on her mother's own past experiences and reflected her own fears. Sally was able to see that the words were not a measure of her worth and did not need to define her. She was also able to see that her mother just wanted the best for her and wanted her to achieve.

I asked Sally if it was acceptable for her to imagine her mother was in the room with us, standing right beside her. She agreed that this was alright. I asked her to imagine what her mother would want to say to her right now.

Tears flowed again as Sally said "She says that she loves me so much and I was always good enough. She said, I'm sorry."

I asked if there is anything Sally needed to say that would allow her to release all the heaviness she had been holding.

Sally smiled, "Yes there is and I'd like a hug from my mum."

I said, "Well you both say what needs to be said and have that hug, take as long as you need and let me know when you are finished."

One or two minutes passed, and sally said, " We are ok now."

After the session Sally revealed that she had always felt judged by her Mother, and since her passing, Sally had wrestled with a heavy feeling of guilt surrounding the tumultuous relationship that they had shared. This insight and others allowed her to understand the impacts of these underlying feelings and assumptions on how she had been feeling in the past two years. It explained the feeling of hopelessness that she had been experiencing knowing that there was nothing she could now do to repair their fractured relationship.

Sally left the session with newfound compassion for herself and a newfound forgiveness for her mother, who she said was just doing the best she could do at the time.

The focus of session three was to reconnect Sally to feelings of joy. She had struggled to remember the last time she felt truly happy. Guided imagery was utilised to help her reconnect with a cherished memory of playing in her mother's garden as a child. She vividly imagined the vibrant flowers, the warmth of the sun, and the laughter that filled the air. This exercise acted as a convincer that it was still possible to experience joy.

Sally reported significant improvements on return to her next session. She reported feeling light in the chest, and the grey had morphed into a sunshine yellow colour. She reported feeling periods of happiness and had more confidence in her workplace. Session four was our final session which focused on future pacing. Sally visualised waking up energised, enjoying her work, and spending quality time with friends. She imagined herself smiling and feeling confident and capable, then importantly she was able to step into this version of herself to get a glimpse of this new reality. As she did this her shoulders dropped further as she released a little more muscular tightness. Tears escaped her and she smiled a broad smile. In that moment Sally stated that she could feel her mother's presence, and she could feel her love flowing through her.

Post-hypnotic suggestions, reinforced these positive images, anchoring them to a simple breathing exercise, of connecting to her exhalation, engaging her parasympathetic nervous system. She was instructed to practice this breath several times a day and employ the technique whenever she felt stressed.

After the sessions, Sally reported that she could now see herself as resilient and capable, rather than a failure. While the grief of losing her mother remained, it no longer consumed her. She started reconnecting with friends, rediscovering hobbies, and even considering a new career path. Sally's journey illustrates the profound potential of hypnotherapy to uncover, heal, and transform.

Depression often convinces its sufferers that change is impossible. Hypnotherapy challenges this narrative by demonstrating that transformation begins within. Through relaxation, exploration, and reframing, individuals can access their inner resources and rewrite their stories.

For Sally and countless others, hypnotherapy offers not just relief but a chance to step out of the shadows and into the light.

Chapter Fifteen

EMBRACING THE PRESENT TO SHAPE THE FUTURE

Having explored the past through the lens of regression therapy in the previous chapter, it is prudent to remember the wisdom of Milton Erickson, who profoundly noted, “People don’t come to therapy to change the past; they come to therapy to change the future.” These words resonate deeply with me, and may remind us all that while understanding the past is essential, our true focus lies in the here and now, as we collectively guide our clients toward a brighter tomorrow.

In our fast-paced world, the present moment often slips by unnoticed. Many clients who come to the consulting room find themselves caught up in ruminations about the past ‘would of’, ‘could of’, ‘should of’ thoughts, or anxieties about the future, all the while missing the richness of the one place where life is actually happening: the present moment.

It is essential that clients come to recognise that the present moment is the only place where true transformation can occur. It is here, and only here, that we hold the power to choose; to repeat familiar patterns and recreate the same outcomes, or to make new, more aligned choices.

This capacity for choice becomes available only through awareness. By teaching clients to cultivate presence, we open the doorway to meaningful decisions, and in turn, to meaningful change.

As a hypnotherapist, I encourage my clients to cultivate a strong sense of present awareness. This practice allows them to step beyond the confines of what they cannot change and embrace what they can. Mindfulness techniques can be a valuable tool in this journey. By learning to observe thoughts, emotions, and bodily sensations without judgement, clients can experience life more fully, fostering resilience and clarity.

Consider the practice of mindfulness as a daily grounding ritual, an invitation to become fully engaged in the present moment. I often guide clients to pause and bring their attention to the breath, noticing the gentle rise and fall of the body. At other times, I invite them to become aware of their senses: to observe what they can feel, see, smell, hear, or taste in that very moment. By engaging all five senses, clients can become anchored in the here and now.

As thoughts arise, they are simply acknowledged and allowed to pass without judgement, as the client's awareness is gently returned to the chosen point of focus. This same practice can be seamlessly integrated into the hypnotic state, where the client's attention may rest on the sound of my voice. Each passing thought is reframed as an opportunity to drift deeper into a state of calm and inner stillness.

Therefore, mindfulness is a valuable practice that can be fully embraced in our moment-by-moment experience both in or out of trance. This is a practice I ask my clients to cultivate and implement in the time between sessions. When clients notice their thoughts drifting into rumination or worry, and deliberately choose to return to the present moment, where none of what they were anxious about is happening, they are empowered to take charge of their current experience, effectively steering their ship into calm waters instead of drifting rudderless into the storm.

This can be as simple as three steps. Step one: I am aware that I'm thinking or feeling that same old thought… again. Step two: asking themselves the question 'Is this helpful?' If I sit with this, will it take me towards where I want to be, or will it fast track me straight back to the problem? If our clients decide that the old thought / feeling or behaviour is not helpful they move to step 3. Let it go. This is achieved by changing their focus to their desired outcome and taking a long slow exhalation, connecting to parasympathetic nervous system and stepping out of stress mode.

This simple, yet profoundly effective practice helps reduce anxiety, restore balance, and create space for insight and self-discovery. As Jon Kabat-Zinn, the pioneer of modern mindfulness-based stress reduction, reminds us: "Mindfulness means paying attention in a particular way: on purpose, in the present moment, and non-judgmentally."

For instance, during a session with a client struggling with overwhelming anxiety and the predictable resulting stress created, we spent time enhancing her present moment awareness. As she focused on her breath both in and out of trance, she began to notice the tension in her shoulders and chest she had been holding could be gently released. By simply acknowledging these feelings without judgment, she was able to soften these muscles simultaneously releasing some of the pressure that was weighing her down . This practice empowered her to feel more in control as she constantly corrected her focus, shifting away from anxiety about the future and toward the choices and the control she had in that moment.

We've explored the importance of being present, of not getting caught in the future, worrying about all the "what ifs" and potential catastrophic outcomes. Equally, we do not want our clients stuck in the past, ruminating over events that cannot be changed. However, it is essential to consider the future, not with fear or avoidance, but in a way that is productive and purposeful. While present-moment awareness lays the foundation for creating calm and safety, cultivating a healthy future focus allows therapy to become not only a process of healing, but one of hope and forward momentum.

I believe without hope; true healing is elusive. Therapy, therefore, is not solely about alleviating current distress; it is about creating a vision for what lies ahead. When clients are encouraged to imagine their desired future, it activates motivation and fosters an internal sense of possibility. According to Snyder's Hope Theory, having a clear goal, combined with the perceived ability to take action and find pathways toward that goal, can significantly enhance psychological well-being. By helping clients envision what is possible, we offer them not only relief, but direction, meaning, and a renewed sense of purpose and possibility.

I often ask my clients to engage in future visualisation exercises during our sessions. By closing their eyes and envisioning their ideal future, clients can articulate their dreams and aspirations with clarity. What does that future look like? How do they feel? What steps can they take to move towards that vision? These questions open a gateway to possibilities and intentions, shifting the focus from limitations to opportunities.

In the hypnotic realm of all possibility, solutions for problems are actively sought. Clients are posed with the question, imbued with suggestion: "When that issue is no longer a concern, how will your life be? What will you feel, do, or think?" Problematic symptoms are explored one by one until the therapist develops a comprehensive understanding of the client's solution-oriented state or goal state, even in cases where the client may struggle to articulate it themselves.

The true power of future direction and a positive future focus is illuminated when clients are encouraged, in a trance state, to embody their future selves. They are invited to feel those emotions and imagine, if only for a moment, that they have already achieved their goals. In that moment, the powerful subconscious mind, which is not literal, does not recognise that this experience is not real, responds instead as though it is.

For example, I worked with a client named Robert who felt stuck in a job that left him unfulfilled. Through future-oriented dialogue that was in direct contrast to his perceived current issues, Robert was able to begin to construct and design a vision of his ideal career, one that involved creativity and an ability to help others.

Robert was invited to get curious about the details as he explored a future version of himself in real time, as if he had already achieved it. Utilising visualisation techniques, he was able to embody that role embracing the feelings and emotions associated with his success. Between sessions Robert was instructed to use self-hypnosis to step into this version of himself each day. Thus, changing his focus from the problem to the solution.

He was educated about the process of neuroplasticity and how creating a positive focus would assist in reshaping his thoughts and feelings and therefore his outcomes. Using cognitive techniques Robert was able to challenge any old limiting thoughts and beliefs as soon as they came into conscious awareness, without lingering in the old problematic habitual way of thinking and feeling. These exercises transformed his perspective from one of resignation to one of empowerment.

By immersing himself in this positive imagery, Robert was able to cultivate a deeper emotional connection to his goal and subsequently take actionable steps to achieve it. This process not only enhanced his motivation but also helped him to rewire limiting beliefs that may have previously held him back.

Hypnotherapy can be a powerful ally in promoting a present-oriented mindset while simultaneously nurturing a future focus. Through guided imagery and suggestion, we can help clients explore their desires and aspirations in a safe and supportive environment. Holistic growth can arise from this dynamic interplay between present awareness and future vision.

As therapists, we can help facilitate this integration, when clients are supported to engage with their past in ways that feel appropriate to them. Some may choose to simply close the door on what has been, while others may revisit and reframe their experiences. Regardless of the approach, all can benefit from actively inhabiting the present while nurturing aspirations for the future. This integrated stance fosters the emergence of an evolving sense of self.

As we encourage clients to focus on the present and the future, it is essential to introduce the concept of self-compassion. Change is rarely linear, and clients may encounter setbacks along the way. I often remind my clients that it's perfectly normal to feel discomfort as they navigate their journey. Embracing self-compassion means allowing themselves to learn from their experiences without harsh self-judgment. It means celebrating progress, no matter how small, and viewing setbacks as opportunities for growth. Each time they become aware they have slipped back into an old pattern, they are aware, and awareness is the key that unlocks the door to change.

In conclusion, let me reiterate, hypnotherapy is a transformative journey that requires both an appreciation for the present moment combined with a hopeful peek into the future. While exploration of the past can certainly be helpful, we must never lose sight of the power of the present moment to guide our clients to embrace their current experiences moment by moment, encouraging them to be creative in envisioning their desired futures.

~

As we come to the completion of this chapter, I invite you once again to reflect on and to remember the powerful words of Milton Erickson, discussed at the beginning of this chapter: "*Clients do not come to therapy to change the past; they come to change the future.*" Our task as hypnotherapists, therefore, is not to dwell in the past, rather to support our clients in reshaping their future by anchoring them in present-moment awareness and nurturing their capacity to envision future possibilities. This can lay the foundation for enduring change, inviting them to step more fully into their goal; the life they are ready to live.

Chapter Sixteen

BREAKING FREE: HYPNOTHERAPY FOR STRESS AND ANXIETY

In today's fast-paced world, stress and anxiety have become commonplace, affecting individuals from all walks of life. The demands of work, familial responsibilities, and societal pressures create a relentless environment where feelings of overwhelm, and unease can take hold. Many individuals find themselves trapped in a cycle of stressful thoughts, often resulting in sleepless nights and a pervasive sense of anxiety that seeps into all facets of everyday life.

To effectively utilise hypnotherapy for relief of stress and anxiety, it is crucial to differentiate between the two. Stress is typically an internal response to an external pressure or challenge which generally triggers the body's "fight or flight" reaction. This is a physiological state that triggers the release of stress hormones such as cortisol and adrenaline. While this response can offer short-term motivation and enhance safety, chronic activation may significantly compromise both physical and mental health (Lazarus & Folkman, 1984)

Unlike a short-term stress response that kicks in when we're facing a clear challenge, anxiety tends to linger for longer, often without any obvious threat in sight. It can present as constant worry, a sense of dread, or feeling on edge for no clear reason. Physically, people might notice a racing heart, tight chest, or tense muscles. If these feelings become overwhelming and start to interfere with everyday life such as work, relationships, or sleep, it could be a sign of an anxiety disorder. In Australia, anxiety is one of the most common mental health conditions, affecting about one in four people at some point in their lives (Beyond Blue, 2024).

Stress is both a biological reaction and a subjective experience, shaped by the complex interplay between body and mind. Neuroscientist Bruce McEwen (2007) describes stress as a state in which the brain orchestrates physiological and behavioural responses to perceived demands or threats. This leads to activation of the autonomic nervous system which triggers the release of stress hormones such as cortisol and adrenaline, priming the body for action, and now you feel stressed.

Psychologists Richard Lazarus and Susan Folkman (1984) emphasise the role of cognitive appraisal, explaining that stress emerges when a situation is perceived as exceeding one's resources for coping. From this view, it is not the event alone that causes stress, but the meaning assigned to it which is influenced by beliefs, past experiences, and perceived supports. This is paramount in the hypnotherapeutic space. Thoughts, focus and beliefs are of prime importance to our client's outcomes. I therefore have a rule that I ask all my clients to remember and embrace that encapsulates this theory, and that is; "what you think, you *will* feel".

Think a happy thought, you feel happy.

Think a sad thought, you feel sad.

Think an anxious thought, you feel anxious.

You see how this works. These are predictable outcomes.

Your amazing body has the capacity to respond to your every thought in an instant, because the subconscious mind cannot differentiate between reality and imagination, and thus responds as though the thought is real. Perceived dangers therefore become reality to your body.

When we explore these two perspectives, we begin to see that stress is a dynamic process: an adaptive, neurological, biological and physiological mechanism that is influenced and moderated by the way we personally interpret and respond to life's challenges.

So, we now understand that both stress and anxiety can arise from the subconscious mind's interpretation of events. This deeper part of the mind stores our ingrained habits and patterns, beliefs, fears and memories, all of which shape how we individually respond to the world around us. As many of you reading this book know, hypnotherapy works at this level, helping to gently reframe perceptions, release unhelpful patterns, and foster a sense of calm, clarity, and empowerment.

Research has shown that the limbic system, which governs emotional responses, plays a critical role in stress and anxiety. Key structures involved include:

1. **Amygdala**: This area acts as the brain's alarm system, detecting threats and triggering anxiety. In those with anxiety disorders, the amygdala may become hyperactive, mistaking benign stimuli for danger. (Hu et al., 2022)
2. **Prefrontal Cortex**: Responsible for higher-order thinking and emotional regulation, the prefrontal cortex's ability to temper the amygdala's responses can be diminished during periods of anxiety (Dolcos, LaBar, & Cabeza, 2004)
3. **Hypothalamic-Pituitary-Adrenal (HPA) Axis**: This system governs the body's stress response by releasing cortisol. Chronic activation of the HPA axis can lead to heightened symptoms of stress and anxiety (McEwen, 2007).
4. **Default Mode Network (DMN)**: This network is responsible for self-referential thought and, when overactive, can

perpetuate cycles of rumination and worry in anxious individuals (Buckner et al., 2008)

Hypnotherapy provides a unique approach to treating stress and anxiety by accessing the subconscious mind, where many emotional responses originate. Unlike traditional therapies that might focus solely on conscious thought processes, hypnotherapy facilitates a deep mental state that enhances receptiveness to therapeutic suggestion.

Hypnotherapy offers several key benefits, including:

- **Initiation of the Relaxation Response**: When deep relaxation is induced in hypnotherapy sessions, the body's parasympathetic nervous system is activated; this is commonly referred to as the "rest and digest" mode. This physiological shift can alleviate the physical symptoms associated with stress and anxiety.
- **Reframing Negative Thought Patterns**: During hypnosis, clients are guided to identify and challenge negative thoughts. This reframing process can transform catastrophic thinking, fostering a more positive and realistic outlook.
- **Accessing the Root Cause**: Hypnotherapy allows clients to explore underlying emotional wounds or traumas in a safe environment. Regression techniques can help reveal the origins of anxiety, enabling clients to release emotional burdens associated with past experiences.
- **Building Resilience**: Suggestions for confidence and inner calm enable clients to cultivate a stronger mental and emotional foundation. By visualising themselves successfully managing stress, clients strengthen neural pathways associated with calm responses, making these reactions more automatic over time.

As hypnotherapists we utilise a wide range of techniques tailored to each client's unique needs and research and literature over many years support these approaches.

Key techniques often include:

- **Progressive Muscle Relaxation (PMR)**: This technique involves systematically relaxing muscle groups to promote deep physical relaxation, often paired with calming suggestions for enhanced effect.
- **Guided Visualisation**: Clients are led to imagine specific peaceful settings, such as a tranquil beach or their favourite childhood place. This imagery can also be used to rehearse positive outcomes in potentially anxiety-provoking situations.
- **Breathing Techniques**: Breathing exercises, such as diaphragmatic breathing, techniques that extend and lengthen the exhalation can be integrated into sessions to help clients regulate their nervous systems and encourage relaxation.
- **Ego-Strengthening Suggestions**: Clients receive empowering affirmations designed to build their self-confidence and resilience, helping them face life's challenges with confidence.
- **Anchoring**: This technique allows clients to establish a physical gesture and link it to a desired emotional state, enabling them to access feelings of calmness during stressful moments.

CASE STUDY: REBECCA'S JOURNEY

Rebecca, a 29-year-old graphic designer, came to the hypnotherapy clinic after years of struggling with social anxiety. On arrival she described a humiliating experience during a high school presentation, after which she developed an intense fear of public speaking and socialising. The symptoms of her anxiety had worsened over time. She now described them as permeating into all areas of her life. The situation had now become debilitating, leaving her feeling unable to cope with work-life demands.

She had been in therapy for several years, having tried psychology-based cognitive-behavioural therapy (CBT) and mindfulness with limited success. Her General Practitioner had prescribed Diazepam (Valium) for occasional use when needed; however, concerned about her lack of progress, and increasing symptomology, he now recommended that Rebecca begin a regular dose of Venlafaxine (Effexor XR), a medication commonly prescribed for anxiety.

Reluctant to commit to daily medication, Rebecca decided to reach out and book an appointment at the clinic. She approached hypnotherapy as a last resort, however after the success of a friend, she held on to a sense of cautious optimism that this could be the answer she had been looking for.

Session 1: Education, building Trust and Creating Safety

In every first session, I begin by educating the client on the intricate connection between the mind and body, emphasising the profound impact our thoughts and our physiology can have on creating immediate chemical and physical changes within us. I introduce tools designed to help clients identify and challenge negative automatic thoughts combined with breath work both to be used outside of sessions. Together we establish a detailed problem state from which we then articulate a vision of their desired solution or goal state when their problem no longer exists.

It's important to note that embedded within this process is a suggestion that fosters an expectation of success, '*when the problem no longer exists*'.

We also engage in a discussion about the critical differences between the conscious and subconscious mind, empowering the client to understand how the body's physiology, biology, and neurology interact in predictable ways. By recognising this, clients can harness this knowledge to formulate a new and more empowering set of instructions, firmly placing them in the driver's seat to select solution-focused alternatives. By consciously choosing different thoughts and by focusing on different emotions, clients naturally experience different outcomes. This empowering principle shifts clients from being passive recipients of their outcomes to being active participants in designing and shaping their future in the present moment.

Establishing a safe and trusting environment where rapport can be fostered is a priority during the first session. I take the time to explain how hypnotherapy works, addressing any concerns about "losing control." Then by using progressive relaxation, which is particularly effective as an induction technique for clients experiencing anxiety or stress, I guided Rebecca into a light trance.

It's important to emphasise that whatever level of trance a client achieves is perfectly fine. It is essential to reassure our clients that they can find success at a level that is right for them in this moment. This reassurance helps alleviate worries such as "It's not working," "Am I doing this right?" or "I can't be hypnotised," as well as any other cognitive distortions that might threaten to disrupt their trance experience.

After an informed introduction to the process, Rebecca was able to experience the soothing effects of hypnosis without distractions. Rebecca was guided to notice how she was able to release any muscular tightness or tension as she surrendered to this moment where she felt safe to relax. She was then able to visualise a safe place. She chose her cosy living room filled with soft light and warmth with her furry companion, her trusted dog, beside her. This image was utilised and called upon in the times between sessions to calm and comfort her when required.

It's essential to recognise that this physical state of trance induced relaxation, may be something our anxious clients have not experienced in a very long time. It is reinforced whilst in trance that this is a state that 'she' has created and can carry with her, or re-enter at any point by challenging her old repetitive thoughts, focusing on her breath, particularly her exhalation and changing her focus to something more pleasing such as her 'safe place' image.

Between sessions she was tasked to be the observer of her thoughts, challenge any old repetitive thoughts without judgement, utilise breath techniques to step out of stress mode and continue to focus on her solution state, actively stepping into it each day as if she had already achieved it.

Session 2: Uncovering the Root Cause

In our second session, I employed regression therapy to explore the origins of Rebecca's anxiety. Whilst in trance, Rebecca vividly recalled the high school incident, remembering her trembling voice, the anxious feelings in her chest and the sound of muffled laughter. At this point, it is essential to establish that this was the first time Rebecca had experienced such feelings, and it was. If Rebecca had remembered a prior event, we would have gone to that event and continued with the same process. It is important to be working with the earliest, or first event for complete resolution to occur, or the symptoms may persist.

Having established that this was the initiating event, we explored the memory through the eyes of her younger self, noting the emotions that were present, the meanings she had assigned to those emotions, and other details of the event. When this self-exploration was fully exhausted, I called upon her older, wiser self. The purpose of this is to allow the current version of herself to float above the younger distressed self, in doing so, allow her younger self to understand what she knows now that she did not know when she was so much younger.

Now armed with the resources and wisdom accumulated over the years, Rebecca was able to reinterpret the events in a way that felt far more relevant and informed. I transcribed her revelations as the session progressed and fed them back to her as therapeutic suggestions when the trance was deepened. Because these were her own words and her own revelations they were easily integrated and accepted by her subconscious mind. Guided reframing was also utilised to help Rebecca see the incident from a new perspective, enabling her to release the long-held shame and fear. She was then future paced to embody living life from her own more solution focused perspective.

Post hypnotic suggestions were given to notice the changes that were occurring every day, and to continue the practices from session one.

Session 3: Anchoring Confidence

The third session focused on all the changes she had been observing and on enhancing Rebecca's calm and confidence. This was facilitated by asking Rebecca to recall a moment when she felt confident and capable.

Rebecca was able to immediately bring such a memory to mind. I invited her to visualise this experience in vivid detail, encouraging her to connect with the emotions she felt at that time, the pride, elation, and sense of accomplishment. She was directed to notice the sounds, the sights, and the sensations of that moment. As she began to engage with this powerful memory, I asked her to pay attention to the positive feelings that arose within her.

I guided Rebecca to anchor these feelings by associating them with a physical gesture. Using a common anchor technique, I suggested that she gently press her thumb and forefinger together while exhaling deeply, creating a tangible link between her mind and body. She was instructed to embody the positive feelings, in the present moment, as she did this several times.

It was suggested that she could create this feeling anytime by pressing the anchor and imagining the success feelings any time she needed to. The repetition of this practiced over time reinforced the connection between the physical action and the empowered feelings. Once she felt fully anchored in this confident state, I gradually guided her back, suggesting that she would retain this feeling as she returned to her everyday life. Through this process, Rebecca not only anchored her confident feelings but also left the session with a practical tool she could utilise whenever doubts threatened to resurface.

Again, she was instructed to continue all the practices from previous sessions on a daily basis, keeping her focus on her goal state.

Session 4: Further future Pacing and building expectation for ongoing change.

The final session centred on noticing the continuing changes Rebecca was experiencing and on noticing how far she had come. As with all sessions noticing these changes in the present and designing the future with a positive expectancy was priority.

Rebecca had an upcoming presentation that she wanted to focus on, so in trance Rebecca associated to and embodied the desired version of herself who can easily and seamlessly give a confident presentation at work, her voice steady and her body relaxed, her mind clear.

This session was recorded so Rebecca could listen to it twice a day leading up to the presentation. This reinforced her ability to easily access this confident state and further embedded suggestions for success. As mentioned in previous chapters repetition is paramount in creating permanent neurological and physiological outcomes. It is also empowering for our clients as they realise that they play an active part in their own success.

Outcome

Over the following weeks, Rebecca experienced significant transformations. She felt at ease in social settings and even volunteered to lead a team meeting, a milestone she once deemed impossible. While occasional nerves persisted, she now had effective tools to manage them.

Hypnotherapy helps clients reclaim their power, teaching them to quiet their minds, reframe fears, and cultivate resilience. For Rebecca and countless others, hypnotherapy offers not just relief but renewal, a chance to break free from the constraints of stress and anxiety, stepping confidently into a life filled with possibility.

In conclusion, harnessing the power of the subconscious mind through the skilful use of hypnotherapy, can create the perfect environment to allow individuals to transform their relationships with stress and anxiety. By addressing the subconscious origins of these challenges, hypnotherapy can allow clients to rewrite their narratives and step into their potential.

As many great Hypnotherapists in the past have stated, 'the answers you seek are already within you'. Hypnotherapy simply helps you uncover them, illuminating the path to personal growth. Through curiosity, exploration, and empowerment, hypnotherapy opens the door to healing, helping clients emerge from the darkness to embrace a brighter future.

In a world that often feels overwhelming, hypnotherapy serves as a reminder that peace is always within reach, one breath, one thought, and one session at a time.

Chapter Seventeen

HARNESSING YOUR INNER STRENGTH: HYPNOTHERAPY FOR SELF-ESTEEM AND CONFIDENCE

Self-esteem and confidence are not innate traits; rather, they are skills we can learn and cultivate over time. These vital aspects of self-perception shape how we interact with the world and respond to life's challenges. Yet, they are often compromised by negative experiences, critical self-talk, or unhelpful beliefs. This chapter explores how hypnotherapy can be a powerful tool for rediscovering your inner strength, breaking free from limiting beliefs, and embracing your authentic self.

When we understand the principles of self-esteem, we see that it reflects how much you value yourself, while confidence pertains to your belief in your ability to perform tasks and face challenges. Both concepts are interconnected; a deficiency in one often affects the other. Dr. Nathaniel Branden, a leading psychologist in self-esteem, emphasised that building self-worth relies on two key practices: living consciously and practising self-acceptance (Branden, 1994).

Hypnotherapy seamlessly integrates these principles by helping clients uncover unconscious barriers, replacing them with empowering beliefs. When we undervalue ourselves or doubt our capabilities, it affects our interactions and choices. Low self-esteem might lead to avoidance of opportunities, while a lack of confidence can result in missed chances for personal and professional growth. The first step toward change involves recognising these patterns and understanding their origins. This is where hypnotherapy shines and provides a powerful modality for self-exploration and transformation.

Hypnotherapy is about reconnecting to your authentic self, free from fear, doubt, and the weight of external, and importantly, internal judgment. By entering a hypnotic state of focused attention, the conscious and judgemental mind can quieten, allowing the subconscious to become more open and receptive to suggestions and insights.

The common benefits of hypnotherapy for self-esteem and confidence include the ability for clients to identify and reframe negative self-thoughts and beliefs, reshaping outdated thoughts and feelings that have held them back. Effective hypnotherapy can reduce the volume of the inner critic's voice by addressing the underlying causes of self-criticism, often rooted in harsh words or impressions from others. Once these issues are brought to light, clients can learn to challenge and replace harsh judgments with kinder, more compassionate self-talk. Enhancing self-compassion and resilience begins with fostering a nurturing relationship with oneself and promoting an inner dialogue built on love rather than criticism.

Hypnotherapy can also help with boosting our client's performance in social or professional situations. Successful outcomes and noticeable changes are natural convincers, as confidence increases, clients often find that they are more willing to engage in social activities and pursue new opportunities.

I doubt you will be surprised to learn that low self-esteem and a lack of confidence often serve as underlying themes in many of our clients' presenting issues. These detrimental factors can impact various aspects of a person's life, from relationships to professional endeavours. Consequently, it becomes essential for therapists to master effective strategies for addressing these presentations during client sessions. By developing a comprehensive understanding of self-esteem and confidence, we can create a supportive environment that fosters growth, empowers clients, and facilitates meaningful change.

According to Ernest Rossi, Dr. Milton Erickson believed that individuals hold the answers within themselves, and hypnotherapy facilitates access to this inner wisdom. It is through this process that clients can unlock their potential and cultivate a healthy sense of self-worth.

CASE STUDY: EMMA

Emma, a 35-year-old teacher, sought hypnotherapy after struggling with low self-esteem for years. Her inner critic constantly told her she wasn't good enough, leading to social anxiety, pervasive self-doubt and a rather large case of imposter syndrome.

During our sessions, we uncovered a belief rooted in her childhood: "I'm not as smart as others." Using regression techniques, we revisited the origin of this belief, unearthing moments that had shaped her self-perception. Through powerful visualisation exercises, Emma practised seeing herself as a capable, confident educator rather than the self-doubting individual she had been conditioned to believe she was.

After six sessions, Emma reported significant improvements in the way she felt about herself and her abilities. The use of journaling and a scaling system had provided her with concrete evidence of her overall progress and allowed her to create a vision for her ongoing success. Emma felt empowered by her newfound insight and began volunteering for leadership roles at school. She felt increasingly comfortable expressing her thoughts and ideas during meetings and more significantly, she started dating again. She now approached relationships with a confidence that she had previously thought was unattainable.

Emma recognised that this transformation was not merely a stroke of luck; it was the result of her commitment to her own personal growth and self-discovery. Even after her sessions were complete, she continued to utilise all the tools she had acquired. She understood that she had achieved her desired outcome, by utilising the tools she had learnt during the sessions. Emma was aware that discontinuing these new practices could easily leave her vulnerable to old habits and patterns reforming and this path of least resistance, could lead her right back to where she began. Therefore, Emma was aware that building self-esteem and keeping it, is not a one-time process.

As part of her therapy, Emma incorporated daily affirmations into her morning routine to maintain her focus on her desired solution state. Each day, she repeated positive statements such as "I am good enough," "I am a competent teacher," "I am successful," and "I feel confident when teaching." It is essential to emphasise that all affirmations should be stated in the present tense, as if they have already been achieved. This approach reinforces their validity and effectiveness, as we remember that the subconscious mind will respond to every thought as though it is real in that moment.

With this in mind, Emma was encouraged to express gratitude for her success, confidence, and competence, behaving as if she had already realised these achievements. This self-hypnotic technique enables her subconscious mind to respond as if these positive statements are reality, thereby instigating instant changes in her body chemistry that align with her thoughts. As a result, Emma began to genuinely feel the emotions associated with her affirmations.

Over time, this practice rewired her brain for positivity, solidifying these empowering thoughts and feelings. By concentrating her attention on affirmations that affirm her worth and capabilities, Emma strengthened her desired outcomes, reinforced her sense of self-worth, and cultivated a positive mindset. As her confidence grew, she found herself better equipped to navigate challenges and grasp opportunities, ultimately transforming her life in meaningful ways.

Journaling was an important practice that Emma employed to reflect on the changes she experienced throughout her hypnotherapy sessions. This technique served as a valuable tool, as it allowed her to document her progress and insights, making it easier to recognise the small changes that might otherwise have gone unnoticed. By regularly recording her thoughts, feelings, and experiences, Emma created a tangible account of her journey towards self-improvement. It provided a structured way to observe the frequency and duration of changed feelings, thoughts, and emotions, ultimately enabling Emma to track her transformations in a measurable manner.

This process not only offered concrete evidence of the positive changes occurring in her life but also fostered a sense of accountability and self-reflection. Moreover, seeing her progress laid out on paper served as a source of encouragement and inspiration, motivating her to continue her journey towards deeper self-awareness and growth.

Research supports the benefits of journaling in the context of personal change. Expressive writing can lead to improved emotional well-being, greater self-awareness, and enhanced problem-solving skills.

By converting her thoughts, feelings and behaviours into words, Emma enhanced her ability to process her experiences, clarify her thoughts, and foster a greater understanding of her own progress.

Between sessions, mindful self-compassion was also employed to reduce self-judgment whenever old thoughts surfaced. This practice allowed Emma to become more aware of her previous negative self-talk and critical inner voice without being harsh on herself. Instead of reacting with self-criticism or suppression, she learned to notice these thoughts with a sense of curiosity and understanding. By acknowledging their presence without judgment, Emma was able to release them, preventing them from having a detrimental impact on her well-being.

Once she recognised and let go of these unhelpful thoughts, the focus of her attention was redirected towards solution-focused intentions. This was often applied as a self-hypnotic activity, even for as little as a minute where she remembered who she was becoming and stepped into that version of herself as a 'reset' of types. This shift encouraged her to concentrate on positive outcomes and strategies for growth, fostering a mindset that embraced possibilities and self-improvement, and encouraged positive neuroplasticity.

By cultivating mindful self-compassion, Emma not only alleviated feelings of inadequacy but also strengthened her ability to approach challenges with resilience and an increased sense of self-acceptance.

She was encouraged to notice moments when she successfully achieved this outcome and to bring her observations to each session for discussion. These instances, along with all other changes, were integrated into her hypnotherapy sessions as positive suggestions that highlighted how things were changing for the better in so many ways, further consolidating her progress at the subconscious level. This is an important point; all changes can be noted and applied as positive suggestions in the hypnotic trance. These observed changes will be readily accepted by the client's subconscious mind when in trance. We then leverage this point to suggest that our client will continue to notice even more changes. In this way we continue to strengthen the client's outcomes.

The above mentioned multifaceted comprehensive approach enabled Emma to recognise the importance of self-kindness and the cultivation of a positive mindset as essential elements in her journey of personal transformation. Ultimately, Mindful Self-Compassion became a cornerstone of her therapeutic practice, facilitating deeper self-understanding and paving the way for lasting change.

As emphasised throughout this book, lasting change occurs through repetition on both conscious and subconscious levels. You may have heard the saying, "Nothing changes if nothing changes."

Conscious change occurs through awareness and the deliberate choice to think, feel, or act differently, and it is essential to incorporate this principle into every successful hypnotherapy session. By providing tools to foster conscious change, clients can effectively rewire their brains and alter entrenched habits that no longer serve them. This process empowers them to take charge of their thoughts and behaviours, leading to meaningful transformations in their lives.

In contrast, subconscious change involves challenging and reframing old, ingrained habits, thoughts, behaviours, and beliefs that may be limiting one's potential, and to see a way forward to a future that is empowered. This aspect of change addresses the deeper layers of the mind, allowing clients to break free from patterns that have persisted over time, often without their conscious awareness. Hypnotherapy is the key that opens the door to access this potential.

When combined, conscious and subconscious change can create a powerful synergy; one that complements the other in such a way that their union yields results far greater than the individual components alone. This holistic approach not only facilitates deeper healing but also fosters lasting growth and self-empowerment, enabling clients to be active in embracing a more fulfilling and authentic life.

By addressing the subconscious roots of low self-esteem and lack of confidence, you can begin to rewrite your narrative and step into your power. Remember, the answers you seek are already within you. Hypnotherapy simply helps you uncover them, as it illuminates the path forward toward realising your authentic self.

Chapter Eighteen

RESTORING REST: HYPNOTHERAPY FOR INSOMNIA

Have you ever wondered why things always seem worse at night?

Well, there are a few very good reasons that this is so. During the day your brain has lots of distractions, but at night your mind turns inward. Stress-balancing hormones like cortisol play a part by naturally dropping in the evening, and when you're tired your emotional resilience is also lower. Nothing is actually worse, it just feels more intense because of how your body and brain work at night, and this cycle of thinking is an influencing factor in why so many people experience insomnia. For those suffering from this affliction, the darkness can transform the night into a battleground where the relentless struggle for sleep unfolds. On one side is the body, yearning for rest, while on the opposing side is the mind, engaged in relentless chatter and often catastrophising thoughts. Who will win, only exhaustion knows.

As the clock ticks past midnight, every second stretches into an eternity, and beds designed for comfort can transform into sites of great frustration. This chronic inability to sleep not only erodes energy but also chips away at the quality of life in the daylight hours, affecting emotional well-being, cognitive function, and physical health.

Many can relate to the anxious buzz that fills their minds as they lie awake, wrestling with worries about work deadlines, family obligations, or an endless to-do list. Its roots often lie in the complex interplay between stress, anxiety, and the physiological systems that regulate sleep. Hypnosis, with its unique ability to quieten the mind and recalibrate these systems, offers a gentle yet powerful remedy for sleepless nights.

In this chapter, we will explore how hypnotherapy addresses the multifaceted causes of insomnia and helps individuals rediscover the healing potential of sleep. Through a combination of neuroscience, therapeutic techniques, and a compelling case study, we will uncover how hypnosis can transform the lives of those trapped in the cycle of sleeplessness.

Insomnia affects millions around the world, presenting in various forms: difficulty falling asleep, staying asleep, or waking up too early without the ability to return to slumber. Perhaps you have experienced those sleepless nights, staring at the ceiling and feeling the weight of exhaustion yet somehow unable to relax into restorative sleep.

While some experience acute insomnia triggered by stress or life events, others endure chronic insomnia that stretches on for months or even years. The impact of insomnia is far-reaching. Sleep deprivation compromises memory, attention, and emotional regulation while elevating the risk of anxiety, depression, and physical conditions like heart disease and weakened immunity.

Despite its prevalence however, conventional treatments such as medication or cognitive-behavioural therapy (CBT) are not always effective or well-tolerated, leaving many searching for alternative solutions.

Hypnosis is uniquely suited to address insomnia because it engages both the conscious and subconscious mind. By inducing a state of deep relaxation and heightened focus, hypnosis helps bypass the critical, overthinking conscious mind, allowing access to the subconscious where habitual thought patterns and emotional triggers reside.

When individuals enter a hypnotic state, they often find themselves enveloped in a comforting sense of peace that resembles the serene states that typically ease them into sleep. This similarity arises from the brain waves associated with hypnosis, which closely mirror the changes that occur as one drifts off into slumber. During hypnosis, the brain predominantly produces theta waves, which are also observed in the early stages of sleep. Theta waves are associated with deep relaxation, creativity, and the subconscious mind, enabling individuals to access thoughts and memories that may be obscured during waking hours.

In this receptive state, individuals can explore the underlying issues contributing to their insomnia, whether those are rooted in stress, anxiety, or unresolved emotional conflicts. This exploration can facilitate profound healing, as it allows for the identification and reframing of negative thought patterns that interfere with restful sleep. By addressing these core issues within a relaxed and focused environment, hypnosis can promote a greater sense of well-being and pave the way for more restorative sleep.

Sleep is a complex process that unfolds in different stages, each marked by unique brainwave patterns. These range from the fast beta waves associated with waking life to the slow, rejuvenating delta waves found in deep sleep. Hypnosis can help facilitate this transition by encouraging a shift from beta to the more relaxed alpha and theta waves, similar to how the brain naturally prepares for sleep.

Chronic insomnia often results from the excessive activation of the hypothalamic-pituitary-adrenal (HPA) axis, which regulates our stress responses. Hypnosis has been shown to reduce cortisol levels and enhance activity in the parasympathetic nervous system, helping to calm the body and counteract the physiological arousal that can interfere with sleep. Additionally, individuals struggling with insomnia often experience an overactive Default Mode Network (DMN), which is linked to excessive worrying and self-referential thoughts. Hypnosis slows down this network, promoting mental calmness and reducing rumination. Finally, hypnosis supports neuroplasticity, the brain's remarkable ability to adapt and reorganise itself. By replacing negative sleep habits and thought patterns with constructive suggestions, hypnosis helps create lasting positive changes in sleep behaviour

Hypnosis offers various tailored techniques to effectively address insomnia, catering to each individual's specific needs. Progressive relaxation is particularly helpful to reduce physical tension by systematically relaxing muscles, signalling sense of safety to the brain that allows it to step out of stress mode.

Techniques designed to notice repetitive unhelpful thoughts are introduced and reinforced through hypnotic suggestion to enable clients to challenge faulty cognitions and release them without judgement. Sleep preparation imagery can also be used to allow clients to conjure a calming inner atmosphere, such as a sense of peace and safety, or a feeling of letting go of daytime thoughts and a feeling of sinking into the comfort of a warm bed, enhancing feelings of comfort and security. Hypnosis can be utilised to help address underlying stress and anxiety, revealing the root causes of insomnia through processes such as regression or reframing techniques. Establishing sleep anchors and routines, like associating a specific breathing pattern with relaxation can aid in creating a consistent pre-sleep ritual, promoting a more restful night.

Post-hypnotic suggestions are also used to instil positive sleep beliefs that influence ongoing behaviours after sessions, such as feeling relaxed and ready for restorative sleep when lying down and promoting a belief and expectancy that sleep will come easily.

CASE STUDY: JULIE

Background

Julie, a 47-year-old marketing executive, sought hypnotherapy after struggling with chronic insomnia for nearly four years. Her sleep issues began during a particularly stressful period at work and persisted long after the stressors had resolved. She described lying in bed for hours, unable to switch off her thoughts, and waking frequently during the night.

Julie had tried sleep hygiene techniques, over-the-counter remedies, and even prescription medications, but her sleep remained fragmented and unsatisfying. She approached hypnotherapy with a mixture of scepticism and hope, eager for a solution that didn't rely on pills.

Session 1: Education, Building Trust and Understanding

In our first session, I explained the role of the subconscious mind in perpetuating insomnia. Julie was relieved to learn that her sleeplessness was not a personal failure but rather a learned pattern her brain could unlearn. Her habit of thinking about 'everything' when she went to bed was identified and the impact of the active brain state or 'day-time-mode' was discussed as a causative factor in keeping her awake.

I guided her through a gentle progressive relaxation exercise, combined with an awareness tool to enable her to release unwanted thoughts and redirect her attention to the sound of my voice as she was being introduced to the hypnotic state.

Upon coming back to full conscious awareness Julie stated that by focusing on her breath and progressively relaxing her muscles, she had been able to experience a level of calm she hadn't felt in years. This session laid the foundation for deeper work.

Julie was instructed to use this cognitive awareness tool to notice all thoughts that were not helpful throughout the daylight hours and to let them go without judgement, take a breath, and focus on her goal state as though she had already achieved it. The repetitive nature of releasing the problem and focusing on the solution, over and over again, would facilitate the process of neuroplasticity, further facilitated in the trance state.

Session 2: Reframing Sleep Associations

Julie had developed a belief that she 'could not' sleep, and this led to a reluctance of wanting to go to bed because she feared the bedtime frustration and failure she had come to expect.

Listening to our client's words is very important. I always say to my clients, in the words of Henry Ford; "If you think you can, you are right" and "If you think you can't, you are right". The powerful subconscious mind won't judge and will respond to whatever you believe to be true, as if it is.

In trance, therefore we worked to reframe her relationship with sleep. Building an expectancy of sleep was based on the body's inner wisdom, and the truism that she has always known how to sleep from the day she was born. I used guided imagery, asking her to picture her bedroom as a comfortable sanctuary, a safe, inviting space where sleep came effortlessly. Positive visualisations were used as she visualised herself drifting off peacefully and waking refreshed. She was asked to associate with the feelings and emotions of a good night's sleep reinforcing these positive associations with each session.

Session 3: Addressing Underlying Anxiety

To get lasting results it is important to identify where the issue began and ensure it has been dealt with. Therefore, session three was a regression session. It was used to take Julie back to the very first time she had experienced the feeling associated with her current problem. Note I did not say with the insomnia, as sometimes it is not what we expect, so it is important to never lead the clients.

Through regression, Julie accessed the initial memory of a pivotal moment in her life: when she stayed up all night preparing for an important presentation early in her career. She would not allow herself to sleep, as she believed she needed every minute to polish this pivotal presentation. Prior to this sleep had always come easily. She realised that her insomnia had begun that very day, as a way of "staying alert" to avoid failure.

This insight allowed her to reframe her insomnia as a misguided solution to a problem that no longer existed. She also saw the purpose of the insomnia originally had been her subconscious mind's attempt to protect her from failure and the feeling she had carried of not being good enough. Employing reframing techniques, we replaced this outdated belief with a new narrative: "I am good enough", "I am successful", "I can trust my body to sleep easily, knowing that I am capable and prepared for any challenge."

Session 4: Establishing Sleep Anchors

We reviewed Julie's progress, and she had been sleeping well between 6-8 hours per night. An increase from 4-5 hours of disrupted sleep on arrival. She had established a new bedtime routine combining healthy sleep hygiene habits. She was actively using therapeutic self-hypnotic techniques to filter unhelpful thoughts, combined with a breath technique that relaxed her even more each time she noticed she had started thinking. All of this was working well.

The breath became her sleep anchor as she created her new effective bedtime routine. It was encouraging to see that her expectation was growing as she noticed all the changes she had been able to implement. As her expectation grew, so did her positive outcomes, which reinforces the previous statement with a real-world example: "Believe you can, you are right!" Julie's simple breathing pattern, focused on the exhalation being longer and slower than the inhalation. This sent a physiological signal to the brain and body that it was safe, and it was time to relax.

This hypnotic session was utilised to build on and reinforce all positive changes that she had made over the past weeks. Post hypnotic suggestions for continuing to notice changes 'even more' each and every day was reinforced.

Outcome

After four sessions, Julie reported significant improvements in her sleep. She fell asleep more quickly, stayed asleep longer, and woke feeling refreshed. Over time, these changes became self-sustaining, and her anxiety about sleep diminished.

This is such an important topic. An inability to sleep adequately has a ripple effect that is far reaching as it sends its tendrils of impairment out in every direction, impacting every aspect of life from our overall physical and emotional health, work life, home life, and everything in between.

Julie's story highlights an important truth: insomnia is rarely an isolated issue. By addressing the subconscious patterns underlying sleep difficulties, hypnotherapy not only improves sleep but also enhances overall well-being. Clients often report greater emotional balance, increased focus, and a renewed sense of vitality.

For those trapped in the exhausting cycle of insomnia, hypnotherapy can offer a lifeline. By quieting the mind, relaxing the body, and rewriting the subconscious scripts that have driven sleeplessness, hypnosis can restore the natural rhythm of rest, empowering our clients to reclaim their nights and, ultimately, their lives.

Chapter Nineteen

HYPNOTHERAPY FOR PAIN MANAGEMENT

Pain is an unavoidable human experience, yet it remains one of the most complex and subjective phenomena to understand and treat. While acute pain serves an essential biological purpose by signalling injury or danger, chronic pain often becomes a debilitating condition that can linger long after the original cause has healed. Persistent, often debilitating pain of this nature can sometimes lead to physical, emotional, and psychological distress profoundly affecting an individual's quality of life.

Traditional treatments for pain management, such as medication or surgery, often focus on the physical aspects of pain, a band-aid of sorts, that often falls short in addressing its psychological and emotional origins. This is where hypnotherapy can offer a powerful and holistic approach. By working with the subconscious mind, hypnotherapy can help individuals identify, manage, reduce, or sometimes eliminate the often unseen, underlying causes of pain. Importantly, it can empower the client to play and active role in their own healing journey.

In this chapter, we will explore how hypnotherapy can be used to address the issue of acute and chronic pain, the techniques used, and its transformative potential for those who feel trapped by their discomfort.

A compelling case study will also illustrate the profound impact hypnotherapy can have on pain management.

First, we must begin by understanding that pain is not merely a physical sensation; it is an intricate interplay of biological signals, emotional responses, psychological interpretations, combined with social and environmental factors.

As we are coming to understand from previous chapters, the brain plays a central role in so many issues our clients experience, pain is no different. This central role affects how pain is perceived and experienced, making it possible to alter the perception of pain through changes in our clients psychological and subconscious processes.

Before we proceed, we must first differentiate between acute and chronic pain in order to address pain management strategies effectively. Acute pain is a short-term response to injury or illness. Its purpose is often in alerting the body that something is not right, a protective mechanism of sorts, designed to prevent further harm. In contrast, chronic pain persists beyond the normal healing period and can occur regardless of any clear underlying cause. This enduring pain may heighten sensitivity within the nervous system, creating a vicious cycle of pain perception and emotional distress (Schmidt et al., 2023).

Hypnotherapy can interrupt this cycle by targeting the subconscious mind, which governs automatic processes like pain perception. Through relaxation, reframing, and healing suggestions, hypnotherapy can help to turn down the intensity of pain, while shifting the individual's emotional response to it. It is also possible to retrain the brain to respond in different ways so that our clients experience comfort where pain once persisted. (Dillworth, Mendoza, & Jensen, 2012)

Hypnosis has long been recognised as an effective tool for pain management, with roots tracing back to ancient healing practices as mentioned in chapter four of this book; *A Brief History of Hypnosis from Ancient Rituals to Modern Healing*. An abundance of more recent research has now validated its efficacy, demonstrating how hypnosis can alter the brain's response to pain stimuli.

Exploring the neurophysiology of the state of hypnosis with the aid of Functional Magnetic Resonance Imaging (fMRI) has revealed several distinct changes in brain activity that may contribute to pain management.

One fundamental change is the altering of neural pathways; in the state of hypnosis the processing of pain signals in the brain is modified. Functional MRI studies have demonstrated that hypnosis reduces activity in areas associated with pain perception, such as the anterior cingulate cortex and the somatosensory cortex.

In addition to altering neural pathways, the state of hypnosis also enhances our ability to shift focus. It therefore helps clients redirect their attention away from pain toward more pleasant or neutral sensations, effectively diminishing their awareness of the discomfort. In most cases, comfort is a sensation they have paid little attention to as the pain focus have been all consuming. As hypnotherapists we know that whatever we focus on, we strengthen. It therefore becomes of prime importance to direct our client's attention once again toward their solution. Furthermore, hypnosis enables emotional reframing; pain is often exacerbated by emotions like fear, anxiety, or frustration. Hypnotherapy addresses these emotions, fostering a calmer and more empowered relationship with pain.

The state of hypnosis can also promote a deep state of relaxation which, when dealing with chronic pain, is crucial because pain often triggers muscle tension that can worsen the presenting pain. By inducing relaxation whilst in a state of hypnosis, our clients can be guided to release muscular tension and alleviate emotional distress, allowing the body to connect to the parasympathetic nervous system, where healing often occurs more effectively.

When exploring techniques to assist our clients suffering from chronic pain, hypnotherapists can utilise a variety of approaches, all of which are tailored to our client's specific concerns and experiences. In this client group however, once again we see the benefit and effectiveness of utilising a progressive muscle relaxation, which can help our clients access a deep state of peaceful comfort and calm that they may not have experienced in a very long time.

By guiding the client into a state of deep physical and mental relaxation, the hypnotherapist creates optimal conditions for pain relief. In fact, many clients initially benefit from this technique alone, as it encourages them to gently focus on the comfort within their bodies. For those who often express, "I always have pain," this approach can serve as a powerful convincer that alternative experiences are possible. Many individuals who have been living with intractable pain have reported that upon emerging from a first session of hypnotherapy that it was the first time that they had not noticed the pain in very long time. To allow our clients to experience this is a powerful convincer that change is possible.

An important point to remember, during the hypnotic state, it is crucial to avoid mentioning pain, as this can redirect the client's focus back to their discomfort rather than creating a sense of comfort and ease. This principle applies not only during hypnosis but also in the conscious state. In fact, I encourage my clients to alter their language surrounding "pain." Their brain is already wired for the pain response, and their subconscious mind has strong associations with this word and can, and will, immediately seek out the pain as soon as it is mentioned. Therefore, I instruct my clients to look for areas of comfort each morning upon waking, rather than instinctively checking in on "how and where" their pain is that day. Most clients find that replacing the word "pain" with terms such as "discomfort" in their self-talk helps to modify their subconscious response.

Direct and indirect suggestions are skilfully utilised in this, and every client group, to assist in the transition from problem state to goal directed living. Direct suggestions such as, "Your sense of comfort is growing each day" or "as you redirect your focus to comfort you can notice an increasing sense of well-being getting stronger and stronger every day." In contrast, indirect suggestions allow the subconscious to interpret the message autonomously, exemplified by phrases like, "You may soon discover so many things are changing in just the way you imagined they would, or perhaps you are already noticing that?" These suggestions play a vital role in acting as convincers, empowering the client's ability to reframe their previous belief and perception of pain, enabling them to experience a degree of relief. (Hammond, 2010).

Visualisation and imagery are also valuable tools to use in this client group. Clients are encouraged to imagine their pain as something perceptible, such as a block of ice melting, an old picture fading, a colour transmuting from dark to light, or a heavy weight being lifted. This imagery helps shift their focus away from discomfort and fosters a sense of control over their condition.

Time distortion is an additional method that alters the client's perception of time to minimise pain awareness. By suggesting that painful moments feel brief and distant while moments of comfort seem prolonged, hypnotherapists can effectively encourage a more positive experience of time during sessions.

It is also helpful to utilise amnesia in these instances, where our clients are reminded of their ability to 'forget to remember' the discomfort, or 'remember to forget, the choice is always yours'. The added double-bind allows an empowered choice, however either way the client is directed away from the discomfort.

I find it helpful to teach my clients breath techniques that they can utilise at any time to step away from stress, which causes activation of the sympathetic nervous system, and enables them to connect to relaxation by activating the parasympathetic nervous system. Each time they do this they are helping their brain neurologically shift by repeatedly creating a calmer response. This state can be anchored to the breath itself, or to a specific gesture such as pressing their thumb and forefinger together while imagining a wave of comfort flowing from the top of their head to the tips of their toes. The anchor can then be utilised outside of therapy sessions to manage discomfort in real time.

As with so many presenting issues, in this client group the significance of repetition as discussed in Chapter Nine: *Unlocking Change: The Impact of Self-Hypnosis and Repetition,* should not be underestimated. Hypnosis is not a magic cure; however, I have observed over many years that clients who achieve the best outcomes are those who fully embrace the principle of repetition. They constantly challenge old, repetitive, unhelpful thoughts and feelings while committing to daily practices to facilitate neuroplasticity and bioplasticity; *'what we think, we feel'* (Aitken. D, 2025). These are the individuals who often experience remarkable results. I fully believe that change is not only possible; under the right circumstances, it is inevitable.

CASE STUDY: SALLY'S JOURNEY TO COMFORT

Sally, a 50-year-old mother of two, came to me seeking help for chronic lower back pain that had plagued her for years. She had undergone years of physiotherapy, chiropractic therapy, hydrotherapy, acupuncture, all with minimal response as her pain, although alleviated for short periods of time, persisted. She had been on pain medications and was now being encouraged to consider surgery. The constant discomfort she experienced daily affected her ability to work, enjoy time with her family, sleep through the night and was now creating a sense of hopelessness and helplessness that was, on some occasions, leading to depression.

Initially sceptical about hypnotherapy, Sally was willing to try anything that might offer relief. She had been referred by a friend who had success for her own issue, and this had shone a glimmer of hope in Sally's darkness illuminating the possibility that perhaps this could work for her too.

During the initial consultation, it was essential to build rapport and establish an expectation for change. We explored her pain history, its impact on her life, and her treatment goals, concentrating specifically on how her life could improve when pain is no longer an issue. It is important to notice that subconsciously this holds an embedded suggestion. This statement builds an expectancy for change which is so very important in clients living with pain who may have otherwise lost hope. Please note, we have not told our client we can cure their pain, as we cannot, we have merely suggested that change is possible.

We discussed the importance of becoming aware of her repetitive thoughts, feelings, and behaviours, and I introduced a technique to help her challenge faulty cognitions and redirect her focus towards her desired outcomes. She was instructed to stop using the word 'pain' instead she was asked to describe her sensation as discomfort. With this in mind we discussed the physiology of the body and mind and how the subconscious mind will respond to our focus of attention and our thought patterns and will strengthen what we choose to focus on. Therefore, the word pain and all its associations, needed to be eliminated from her dialogue and her focus of attention needed to be redirected.

I explained the process of hypnotherapy, detailing how the brain and body work together in powerful ways to produce outcomes, whether positive or negative, based on the instructions we are creating. While we acknowledged that hypnotherapy might not resolve the underlying cause of her discomfort, its origin being unknown, it could certainly assist her in managing and reducing her perception of it.

In the first hypnotherapy session the focus was on progressive relaxation and introducing Sally to the hypnotic state. We had previously scaled her 'discomfort' which Sally noted as a constant 8/10. I guided her into a deep state of calm, using suggestions to help her body release tension. Sally found it difficult to let go, however by the end of the session, she stated feeling more relaxed than she had in months, though her pain level remained high at a 7/10. It was reinforced that even this was a success, as change can manifest in small degrees.

Sally was instructed to listen to a home recording of a progressive muscle relaxation with suggestions for noticing even more comfort each day. She was also asked to become very aware of her inner narrative and continue to challenge any thoughts that were not helpful. Her next session was one week later.

In our second session, Sally reported feeling hopeful. She had had moments where she had not noticed the 'discomfort' and she was pleased with this. She had diligently been doing her home tasks and was doing the progressive muscle relaxation twice daily.

We began further reframing Sally's perception of her discomfort. Sally had described the sensation in her back as a 'pulsating red fireball'. Using guided imagery, I asked her to visualise the red fireball in her lower back, I then referred to her own inner knowing by asking her to identify what would work best to soothe it. Sally wanted to pour ice cold, blue water on it to put the fire out and create more comfort. Using guided imagery, this is exactly what she did. The pulsating fireball extinguished momentarily, leaving a much smaller area of glowing embers. She poured more ice blue water on it to further comfort the area, and it was suggested that she could do this anytime she needed to maintain or increase the comfort. Her home tasks continued as for session one, with this additional instruction. Again, here it is important to note the focus was on increasing the comfort, not diminishing the discomfort. Words are powerful and focus is paramount in our client's achieving optimal outcomes.

By the third session, Sally felt more in control of her comfort levels. Although her discomfort was still experienced as an 8/10 on some occasions, it was more commonly now floating between a 6-7/10. She did not focus on this and immediately extinguished the fire whenever she felt it was required and had discovered that changing her language, and her expectation for comfort to be felt in the area, had changed her day-to-day experience.

She expressed that the old unhelpful thoughts continued but not as often as she chose to no longer sit with them. We discussed again the principles of neuroplasticity, and how the brain will go through a process of synaptic pruning when it notices we are no longer running old patterns of thoughts or focus of attention. An outcome of this is that the old thoughts will cease to be sent by the brain when it is observed that they are given no airtime. The brain in its wisdom will take its energy, and its neurotransmitters, to other functions that are thought to be more important, the ones we continue to give great attention to.

In the following session, we embarked on a journey to explore the origins of Sally's discomfort. Regression techniques were employed to uncover the emotional factors that may have contributed to her distress. Through this process, Sally accessed a traumatic memory she had long since forgotten on a conscious level. She recalled a time when she was pregnant and entangled in an abusive relationship, where she had endured physical violence at the hands of her intoxicated husband.

In this painful memory, she vividly remembered turning her back on her husband in an attempt to shield and protect her unborn child. As she crouched to defend herself, he struck her repeatedly on the back. Although this did not cause physical damage to her spine, years later the psychological scars from losing the pregnancy lingered with her to this day. She carried a subconscious guilt, believing it was her fault and that she should have done more to protect her child.

Additionally, Sally shared her later struggles with infertility, expressing that she felt she was being punished for not being able to safeguard her unborn child. She felt a part of her had sabotaged her attempts to conceive again. Processing, reframing, and releasing this memory provided her with the emotional relief she needed, allowing her to mourn for her lost child and the trauma she had internalised.

She wept for the child she would never know and importantly for the battered woman she had once been. This abreaction allowed her to begin the process of release of that which she had been holding onto for so long. By the end of the session, she felt emotionally spent yet liberated, sensing that a deep weight had been lifted from her shoulders.

Sally was encouraged to be gentle with herself between sessions and to anticipate feeling emotional during this time. She was advised not to judge her feelings but to allow all thoughts and emotions to flow naturally, recognising that this is a normal part of processing her grief and trauma. Additionally, she was reminded to utilise the tools she had learned to find stillness and calm by connecting to her breath.

After four sessions, Sally reported a significant reduction in both the intensity and frequency of her pain, now describing it as a 2/10, and at times, it was hardly noticeable. She was able to resume normal daily activities that she had previously avoided, such as working, gardening, and walking along the beach. Most importantly, she expressed a renewed sense of hope for the future.

This case study is just one example of how hypnotherapy can transform the experience of pain, showcasing its profound benefits. Many clients find they can reduce their reliance on medication, lowering their dosage of painkillers or even stopping them altogether in consultation with their doctor, which leads to fewer side effects and overall better health. Hypnotherapy can also help clients re-engage with activities they once enjoyed, fostering a renewed sense of normalcy and fulfilment in their daily lives.

As clients gain invaluable tools to manage their discomfort independently, they experience a sense of empowerment which can diminish feelings of helplessness and hopelessness that may lead to depression. Additionally of great importance as seen in this case study, addressing the emotional aspects of pain can bring significant relief, allowing clients to cultivate a greater sense of peace within themselves. Ultimately, these transformative effects not only alleviate pain but also enhance overall well-being, illustrating the powerful potential of hypnotherapy in pain management.

Pain, while a deeply personal experience, does not have to define a person's life. Hypnotherapy offers a compassionate, empowering, and effective way to manage pain by addressing its physical, emotional, and psychological dimensions. Through relaxation, reframing, and emotional healing, hypnotherapy can help clients find relief where other treatments may have failed. It reminds us that even in the face of chronic pain, there is always the potential for comfort, resilience, and transformation. This journey is not just about alleviating discomfort; it is about reclaiming one's life and embracing a future filled with possibility.

The future of hypnotherapy for the use of managing pain is promising. As research continues to validate the effectiveness of hypnotherapy for pain relief, it is increasingly being integrated into mainstream medical settings. Hospitals, cancer treatment centres, and chronic pain clinics are recognising its value as a complementary approach. Also, the non-invasive nature of hypnotherapy makes it a compelling option for individuals seeking alternatives to conventional treatments for pain management. Its ability to address the mind-body responses aligns with the increasing emphasis on holistic healthcare. With ongoing advocacy and education, hypnotherapy has the potential to become a cornerstone of pain management, offering hope and relief to millions around the world.

Chapter Twenty

HARNESSING THE POWER OF HYPNOTHERAPY TO ALLEVIATE IRRITABLE BOWEL SYNDROME

Irritable Bowel Syndrome (IBS) is a complex and often debilitating gastrointestinal condition characterised by abdominal pain, bloating, and irregular bowel habits. It affects an estimated 10-15% of the global population and significantly impacts individuals' quality of life, yet its underlying causes often remain elusive.

Traditional medical approaches, including dietary modifications and medications, can be essential for symptom management for some individuals, however there is a growing body of evidence that supports the effectiveness of hypnotherapy as a valuable complementary treatment.

Central to understanding IBS is the concept of the gut-brain axis: a bidirectional communication system that links the gastrointestinal tract and the central nervous system. This intricate connection helps explain why stress and emotional states can exacerbate IBS symptoms. Chronic stress, anxiety, and unresolved emotional trauma can disrupt gut motility, alter the gut microbiome, and heighten pain perception. (Häuser, W., 2024).

Hypnotherapy utilises the gut-brain axis to influence and reframe the body's response to stress, restoring harmony between mind and body.

By addressing the psychological triggers and stressors associated with IBS, hypnotherapy can significantly reduce symptom severity and improve overall well-being.

Hypnotherapy for IBS, often referred to as gut-directed hypnotherapy, employs specific techniques designed to target the gut-brain connection. These sessions are tailored to the individual's unique symptoms, emotional triggers, and underlying stressors.

IBS often thrives in a state of heightened stress. Thus, once again our clients are benefited by being guided into a state of deep hypnotic relaxation using methods such as progressive muscle relaxation (PMR) and guided imagery. This relaxed state reduces the activation of the sympathetic nervous system and promotes a parasympathetic response that aids in digestion and calms the gut.

At this point we are reminded of the stress responses' impact, discussed in chapter 16; *Breaking Free: Hypnotherapy for Stress and Anxiety.* Stress plays a crucial role in our overall health, particularly concerning the gastrointestinal tract. When we encounter stress, our body activates the "fight or flight" response, triggering a cascade of physiological changes, including the release of stress hormones like cortisol. This reaction can disrupt gut motility, alter digestive processes, lead to increased inflammation, bloating and even affect the balance of gut bacteria.

Due to this 'gut impact' stress reduction is a crucial therapeutic focus for these clients. Cognitive techniques are employed in the conscious state to help clients challenge stressful thoughts and emotions, alongside tools designed to disengage from stress or sympathetic nervous system activation. Positive outcomes are integrated into the hypnotic sessions, reinforcing clients' abilities to create change and concentrate on their desired state. A better understanding of the mind-body connection empowers individuals to adopt stress management techniques that enhance both mental and gut health, ultimately improving their overall well-being.

As we have established, the subconscious mind responds to our every thought. We can harness this physiological response to achieve the desired outcomes for our clients. One effective approach is to encourage clients to visualise their gut functioning normally and comfortably. They may imagine their digestive system as a gently flowing river or a balanced, efficient system. The specific imagery doesn't matter, as long as it is meaningful to our clients.

The message is clear, and our clients are reminded that their bodies inherently know how to function optimally when provided with the right conditions to thrive. This practice helps retrain the subconscious mind to associate a calm inner environment with normal gut function, fostering a sense of autonomy and control in the clients.

Heightened pain sensitivity is often seen in clients who struggle with IBS. Hypnotherapy can be employed to help alter the brain's interpretation of these pain signals. For instance, clients may be guided to visualise a control room where they imagine a "dial," "scale," or "switch" that they can manipulate to reduce their pain. This technique empowers them to adjust their discomfort, decrease sensations, or even turn them off altogether, whilst simultaneously increasing the comfort control.

Unresolved emotional trauma can significantly exacerbate IBS symptoms. Hypnotherapy provides a safe space for clients to explore these triggers, enabling them to process and release emotional burdens that often manifest physically. Techniques such as age regression, parts therapy, and Rewind Technique can help alter the emotional response associated with traumatic memories by reframing how the brain perceives these events. This process can notably reduce feelings of anxiety, fear, and distress, promoting healing and emotional release. Additionally, safely executed gestalt conversations with perpetrators can allow clients to express what they could not articulate at the time, further addressing the remnants of trauma. By working through these emotional challenges, clients can alleviate symptoms and foster overall healing and well-being.

A growing body of research underscores the effectiveness of hypnotherapy in managing IBS symptoms. As far back as 1987, A landmark study by Whorwell et al. revealed that gut-directed hypnotherapy led to significant reductions in abdominal pain, bloating, and bowel dysfunction in patients with IBS, with lasting improvements observed even after the treatment concluded. More recent systematic reviews and meta-analyses support these findings. Hypnotherapy has been shown to be a highly effective treatment for IBS, often surpassing other psychological therapies. Gut-directed hypnotherapy has been shown to not only alleviate symptoms but also enhance quality of life whilst reducing levels of anxiety and depression among individuals with IBS.

There has now been so much good quality research on this topic that we are currently seeing the implementation of gut directed hypnotherapists in large tertiary hospitals across Australia such as the Alfred Hospital in Victoria, which operates a Functional Gut Clinic offering gut-directed hypnotherapy along with various treatments for conditions like IBS. It is reassuring to notice that the clinic adopts a multidisciplinary approach, providing clients access to dietitians, psychologists, and hypnotherapists.

While hypnotherapy is a powerful tool for managing IBS, it can be more effective when integrated into a holistic treatment plan. Dietary modifications, along with lifestyle changes such as regular exercise and mindfulness practices can enhance the effects of hypnotherapy and contribute to overall well-being.

We all bring something unique to our sessions with clients, and I encourage everyone to leverage their expertise to create a distinctive therapeutic experience. I have worked extensively with clients struggling with IBS, drawing on my clinical expertise to inform my approach. My background in healthcare, combined with my skills as a clinical hypnotherapist, allows me to tackle IBS from a holistic perspective.

In each new client session, I start with a detailed exploration of their lifestyle factors, emotional triggers, and symptom patterns, examining any beliefs and unhelpful thought processes that may contribute to their condition. This thorough understanding enables me to tailor hypnotherapy interventions that address both the physical symptoms and the psychological factors unique to each individual. I emphasise the potential of mind-body self-empowerment practices that place clients in the driver's seat of their own journeys.

Through hypnotherapy sessions, I guide my clients not only in alleviating their symptoms but also in developing sustainable tools for self-regulation and resilience. This dual focus on symptom relief and emotional well-being has helped many of my clients regain control over their lives, allowing them to reconnect with a sense of balance and vitality.

Once again, we are reminded that the body is not simply a collection of disconnected systems, but a holistic, integrated whole. Nurturing one aspect, whether through physical care, mental focus, or emotional healing, naturally elevates the functioning of the entire system. In this way, mind and body work synergistically, generating a capacity for health and resilience that far exceeds what each element could achieve on its own. Each dimension continuously interacts with and influences the others, sustaining a dynamic state of balance.

As hypnotherapists, we must recognise that a presenting issue can never be reduced to isolated symptoms. The reality is far more complex. IBS is not a condition that affects only the gut, but also the mind and emotions. Hypnotherapy offers a unique, evidence-informed approach to addressing the underlying patterns of IBS, providing relief that extends beyond basic symptom management. By calming the gut–brain axis, reframing the experience of pain, and resolving emotional triggers, hypnotherapy empowers individuals to reclaim control of their health and significantly improve their quality of life.

As a compassionate, non-invasive therapy, hypnotherapy holds immense potential for those seeking relief from IBS. When integrated with other therapeutic approaches, it can foster lasting change and help clients rediscover a life less constrained by the challenges of this condition.

Chapter Twenty-One

UNLOCKING POTENTIAL: HYPNOTHERAPY FOR CHILDREN

In my practice, I commonly see children who are experiencing a variety of emotional concerns that often present physically. Symptoms as varied as abdominal pain and stomach upsets to behavioural issues such as school avoidance, separation anxiety and general fears related to everyday life are not uncommon. Unsurprisingly, these occurrences have increased significantly since the Covid-19 pandemic, with many children now needing to learn additional skills in the form of therapeutic tools to help them navigate the often confusing and sometimes frightening post-pandemic world they find themselves in.

The good news is that children are fantastic subjects for hypnotherapy, and as hypnotherapists, it is essential that we engage their creative imaginations. By tapping into their childlike ability to envision vibrant scenarios, such as colourful dragons, flying spaceships, and time travelling machines that can take them out to a brighter future. We utilise these imaginative creations as perfect vehicles for transformation, enabling the child to develop resilience and confidence and a sense of safety in their everyday lives.

Children generally navigate the world with boundless imagination, curiosity, and an innate ability to daydream. However, life's challenges, be they academic, social, emotional and yes, even Pandemics, can often lead young minds to utilise this very same imaginative potential to take them directly to their worst and most catastrophic imaginings. This transformation can rapidly overwhelm developing brains, drawing them into the daunting landscape of their deepest fears, where every dread feels frighteningly real.

Hypnotherapy, with its emphasis on creativity and subconscious communication, offers a gentle, non-invasive approach to help children overcome such fears, which are often unknowingly of their own creation, and direct them onto a path toward self-empowerment, no matter what their age.

In this chapter, we will explore why hypnotherapy can be particularly effective for children and how these unique techniques can foster resilience, emotional regulation, and self-confidence. Jason's journey, a case study of a 12-year-old struggling with anxiety and academic pressures, will illustrate the transformative potential of hypnotherapy in a child's life.

Throughout my years as a hypnotherapy and counselling tutor, as well as a clinical supervisor, the question I often encounter is whether hypnotherapy can be effectively employed with young children. My response is always a resounding yes. However, is it always successful? Perhaps not. There is no singular remedy that works for everyone. Just as with any client, we must approach each child as an individual, taking into account their natural receptiveness and vivid imaginations, which make them ideal candidates for hypnotherapy.

As with adults, we often work with resistance in this client group, integrating it into our approach. It's important not to anticipate that your young client will sit still; they most likely will not. Expect your younger clients to wiggle and squirm, this is perfectly acceptable. Utilise it, normalise it, and work with it. You might say, "you know I find that my clients who wriggle about get the best results" or "It's so good to see that there is a part of you that knows how to get into the most comfortable position as you settle in to listen to the story I'm about to tell you."

The other important thing I will say when working with children, is keep your sessions short. You will definitely lose them if the session goes too long. I recall a young child who kept announcing to me how many minutes of the session were left to go. I said, I understood that he may not have wanted to be here on such a beautiful day, and that I would rather be at the beach too, but since he was here and we had 17 minutes to go, why not use that time to good effect so he could feel better faster and when he did he wouldn't need to come back. The embedded suggestion was that he could get better quickly, or it could take as long as he wanted it to take. I was happy to see him for many more sessions if that was his choice. In that moment, a seed was planted; he had the power to choose, whether he would experience quick improvement and therefore, shorten his time with me, or allow his journey to take longer. He fully utilised the remaining 17 minutes and only required one further session.

When we begin a session with a child it is important to build rapport and create a safe, judgement-free environment. We begin by discovering their interests. What do they love? Who are their heroes? What movies captivate their imagination? What books do they enjoy? Who are their favourite sports figures, and what do they admire about them? We explore their movements, their friendships, and even the delightful quirks of their pets, their names and the amusing antics that make them laugh. This information enriches our connection and helps establish a foundation for building their self-esteem. It fosters the creation of a safe space where we can indirectly challenge any subconscious or unspoken beliefs by highlighting experiences and truisms that contradict those beliefs.

By entering the child's world with genuine interest in their hobbies, fascinations and activities, the therapist has the ability to create a more engaging and personalised experience. When a therapist takes the time to understand what excites a child, they can utilise these interests within therapeutic metaphors and stories, which enhances the effectiveness of the hypnotherapy sessions. For instance, using a familiar character from a child's favourite movie, or a loved sporting champion as a guiding figure in a metaphor, therapy can become more relatable, and engagement is encouraged.

I also find it beneficial to gather insights from parents before the session. This way, I can understand the child's context without putting them on the spot or without the often-undesirable action of discussing parental concerns in front of the child, which may result in the child feeling pre-judged by the therapist before therapy even begins.

I recall a particular instance with a child who struggled with bullying. This child's mother informed me that her daughter had declared she would respond with "no comment" if I asked her anything. Pre armed with this information, rather than diving into therapy immediately, I diverted our conversation to something light-hearted, complimenting her on her lovely jumper. For several minutes, we chatted about it, after which I then inquired about her wellbeing since our last session, her response was minimal as expected. Being pre-warned, I recognised her resistance and normalised it by saying that I didn't feel much like talking today, matching her state and normalising her feelings, I then suggested we go outside to feed the alpacas, an idea she eagerly embraced.

Through the Illusion of seemingly escaping therapy, I was able to further build rapport whilst engaging her imagination in creative ways. We were able to explore the topic of bullying indirectly by discussing the 'pecking' order within the alpaca group and explored the resilience of individual members of the group using stories and metaphors related to the alpacas and their interactions. This style of waking hypnosis proves to be immensely beneficial with children, as it taps into their innate ability to engage in storytelling and allows for unspoken parallels to be drawn, assisting the child to make sense of their own world. Although I am aware that most of you will not have an alpaca family outside your office door, I would suggest utilising anything that you do have to achieve the same result. Get creative, you may be surprised at how well story, metaphors and indirect suggestions can work with children.

Children spend a considerable amount of their time in their subconscious mind, a space that plays a vital role in their development and learning. It is within this realm that experiences, feelings, and memories are stored, shaping behaviour and thought patterns often without their conscious awareness. Research indicates that children's brains are especially active in this subconscious state, particularly during play and imaginative activities, which are crucial for both cognitive and emotional development.

Engaging in imaginative play allows children to process their experiences and make sense of the world around them. Through these creative activities, they explore their emotions and cultivate problem-solving skills to effectively navigate their complex environment. This interaction with their subconscious leads to the formation of beliefs and attitudes that will influence their future interactions and emotional responses.

In this context, hypnotherapy emerges as a valuable tool, leveraging children's natural suggestibility to address various challenges. The unique suggestibility of a child's subconscious mind makes it particularly receptive to positive affirmations and reframing techniques. This heightened sensitivity enables hypnotherapy to effectively confront limiting beliefs and fears, offering a safe and supportive space for exploration without the threat of judgment.

Many children struggle to articulate their feelings verbally, and hypnotherapy's gentle nature helps them navigate this emotional terrain with greater comfort. Engaging strategies such as storytelling, guided imagery and somatic work and metaphors resonate deeply with young clients. For instance, introducing a narrative about a courageous Alpaca, can help a child relate to and understand their own fears in a relatable, non-threatening manner.

Storytelling and guided visualisation serve as powerful therapeutic tools when working with children, fostering engagement and imagination in a way that traditional methods may not achieve. Stories have a natural ability to captivate children's attention, allowing them to explore complex emotions through relatable narratives. By incorporating elements from a child's favourite books or films, therapists can enhance the therapeutic experience, making it more familiar and engaging.

When we utilise guided visualisation in our narratives, we invite the child to immerse themselves in empowering scenarios. Children might envision themselves exploring a magical forest or becoming a superhero who overcomes challenges or defeats the enemy. We may weave beloved characters or storylines into these visualisations making the process more relatable to the child. In these ways hypnotherapy with its non-invasive approach empowers children to harness their inner strengths, allowing them to overcome obstacles independently and foster a sense of control over their circumstances. This therapeutic method aligns seamlessly with children's developmental needs, effectively supporting them in addressing issues such as anxiety, sleep disturbances, phobias, and confidence deficits, all while respecting their unique stages of growth.

CASE STUDY: JASON'S JOURNEY

Jason, a bright and imaginative 12-year-old boy, was referred to hypnotherapy by his mother, after his school counsellor could not help him with his struggles with severe anxiety. The anxiety manifested in physical symptoms, including stomach aches, trouble sleeping, and a reluctance to attend school. The source of his distress was rooted in the increasing academic pressures of starting high school and a profound fear of disappointing his parents. Despite their constant reassurances, Jason had internalised the belief that he wasn't smart enough.

Jason did not enjoy traditional counselling, he found it difficult to express his emotions verbally, leading his parents to seek out hypnotherapy as an holistic approach in hopes of helping him find the relief he desperately needed.

Session 1: Building Trust and Setting the Stage

The first session focused on creating rapport with Jason and making the process enjoyable and non-threatening. I began with light conversation about his favourite hobbies, specifically his passion for space exploration and admiration for astronauts.

Using guided imagery, I led Jason into a gentle trance by asking him to visualise floating through space in a comfortable rocket ship. As he drifted deeper, I introduced a calming image of stars twinkling around him, each representing a worry he could either release into the vastness of space or increase the thruster to move away from them. Choosing the thruster option, Jason noticed how each time he engaged the thruster the worries would burn up and disappear leaving a warming glow behind him. This imagery allowed Jason to get a sense of control over the previously persistent worrying thoughts. He was then asked to imagine his favourite astronaut sitting next to him and I asked Jason what this experienced astronaut would do if a problem arose. Without hesitation Jason said he would 'work the problem' until he found a solution. I then asked Jason to fly through space with his mission commander by his side and together they could 'work the problems' to find permanent solutions to all those worries, as all good astronauts have to do from time to time. At the end of the session Jason described feeling "lighter and more relaxed."

In the second session, we delved into Jason's feelings of not being good enough. I utilised regression to ask Jason the ride his spaceship back to when he first felt that feeling. He once again co-piloted with his favourite astronaut, so he felt completely safe. He floated above a memory of himself when he had failed a maths test, on the same day his brother brought home a sporting award and an 'A' on his recent test. As his parents praised his brother, Jason recalled feeling like he wasn't ever going to be as smart or as good as his brother, who was three years older than him.

We then flew the spaceship to observe his best friend, who had a brother who was two years older than him. Jason was able to understand that his younger friend could not be expected to know what his older brother knew, because his older brother had been learning for two years longer. He was also able to see how his friend's parents loved him even though he didn't know as much as his brother, yet.

I then encouraged Jason to imagine himself as a rocket ready for launch, preparing to explore the wonders of space. However, just like every rocket has its own design and launchpad, some rockets lift off quickly, while others take their time to gather energy before soaring into the stars. Regardless of when they launch, each rocket is precious and adds its own unique adventure to the universe.

Through this metaphor, Jason began to understand that his worth was not tied to his immediate achievements but rather to his unique qualities as a person. Post-hypnotic suggestions reinforced this belief, helping him internalise, "It's okay to grow at my own pace."

The third session focused on building on all the changes that Jason was experiencing and building his confidence and expectancy for ongoing positive outcomes. Continuing to draw on his fascination with space and astronauts, I once again asked him to board the spaceship where he was able to experience successful problem solving as he imagined himself as a daring space explorer successfully navigating space challenges, piloting his ship through an asteroid field to safety by using his inner wisdom and courage. During this and all sessions Jason was instructed to connect to his breath, which allowed him to stay calm under fire and allowed him to think clearly whenever required.

On Jason's fourth and final session, he entered the room with a large smile on his face, walking tall with a confident body language. He happily told me how he had got ten out of ten for his recent maths test. He stated he was using his thruster and burning up all unhelpful thoughts and using his breath tool each day whenever he needed it. We once again entered the spaceship and flew it out to the future to witness his future success and his newfound sense of confidence and resilience. He saw himself walking to school feeling calm and ready to learn, confidently interacting with his peers and teachers, and completing his assignments. His expectation was now one of success. He stated if he failed, he would be able to learn something he did not know, and he would 'work the problem' until he did.

Over the course of four sessions, Jason experienced significant improvements. His stomach aches subsided, he slept more soundly, and he no longer resisted going to school. Teachers observed a positive shift in his behaviour, and he was participating more in class.

Jason's parents were thrilled to see their son smiling again. They reported that he had even started using his "space explorer" visualisation technique before tests, helping him stay calm and focused.

In conclusion, children have an extraordinary capacity for growth and adaptation. Hypnotherapy speaks the language of their subconscious mind and engages them through shared interests, empowering them to overcome challenges, build confidence, and discover their inner strength.

For Jason and countless other children, hypnotherapy can offer not only relief from a presenting concern, but a pathway to ongoing resilience that can last a lifetime. By tapping into their inherent creativity and imagination, children can approach life's challenges with courage and curiosity, fostering a healthier emotional landscape for their future.

Ultimately, hypnotherapy represents a transformative approach that addresses immediate concerns while cultivating long-term emotional intelligence and effective coping strategies. It serves as a valuable resource for parents seeking effective ways to support their children through life's difficulties, enabling them to thrive and realise their full potential.

Chapter Twenty-Two

THE POWER OF HYPNOTHERAPY IN OVERCOMING INFERTILITY

As a nurse and midwife with over 20 years' experience in infertility nursing and IVF, this topic is very close to my heart. With further study and clinical experience, I have come to recognise how much control we possess over the natural functions of our bodies. One of my key messages to clients is the importance of communicating with the body in a language it understands. One very important step in this process involves using awareness and therapeutic tools and practices to activate the parasympathetic nervous system, allowing individuals to access a state of calm. This approach is crucial for our clients who may then correct their path away from stress toward calm whenever their sympathetic nervous system has been incorrectly activated. This principle forms the cornerstone of my work with clients facing infertility.

Infertility can be one of the most emotionally challenging and isolating experiences a person or couple may endure. The journey is often marked by fear, frustration, and profound vulnerability. While advancements in medical science provide various interventions, such as IVF and other assisted reproductive technologies (ART), the emotional and psychological toll of infertility frequently remains unaddressed. Here, hypnotherapy, as part of a complementary mind-body approach, offers significant promise.

During my time as an IVF Nurse and patient care coordinator, I was involved in every stage of the fertility journey, from initial consultations where education was key, to coordination of diagnostic testing, doctor and psychology appointments, cycle monitoring via blood testing and ultrasonography, pre-theatre instructions, medication timing, embryo transfer information, post-treatment care right through to pregnancy test and everything in-between. And believe me there is so much *in-between*. Throughout the process, I consistently noticed that, while medical science offered critical solutions, many patients struggled with the *in-between* of overwhelming anxiety, feelings of inadequacy or guilt and the overall emotional burden of their experiences. Sadly, many also faced dealing with the *in-between* on their own, as they often told no one of their journey. Consequently, these challenges, combined with the financial burden of infertility treatment often overshadowed the joy of planning a family. This realisation inspired my transition into counselling and finally clinical hypnotherapy, equipping myself with further knowledge and skills which would allow me to address the psychological aspects of infertility patient care.

When dealing with infertility clients it is important to cultivate a safe and nurturing environment where clients can explore their feelings openly. I utilise a combination of guided imagery, relaxation techniques, and positive suggestion to help clients process their emotions and regain control over their experiences. My dual expertise in this area has taught me the importance of bridging the gap between the physical and emotional dimensions of infertility, to provide truly comprehensive holistic support.

It is important to recognise that every journey to parenthood is unique. We must therefore take the time to listen to each individual's or couple's story, tailoring our approach to meet their specific needs. This personalised support fosters trust and creates a strong therapeutic alliance, essential for healing.

My sessions are informed not only by a deep understanding of reproductive medicine but also by an intuitive ability to guide clients towards emotional resilience and empowerment. I aim to instil hope, encouraging clients to visualise their desired outcomes and embrace the possibilities that lie ahead. This unique combination of medical insight and emotional guidance makes this approach both holistic and profoundly effective, offering hope and healing to those on the path to parenthood.

Ultimately, our goal is to help clients reclaim their emotional well-being and navigate their fertility journeys with confidence. By addressing both the mental and emotional challenges associated with infertility, we can foster a healthier, more balanced approach to this deeply personal experience. This enables us to create a supportive pathway towards the dreams of parenthood that our clients hold dear.

Given that we can all acknowledge that the infertility journey is inherently stressful on many levels, as detailed in my book *"Sarah's Story, Life after IVF,"* reducing it is a key factor in working with this group. As mentioned many times throughout this book the relationship between the mind and body is a powerful one which has been extensively documented with numerous studies demonstrating the effects of psychological stress on physical health, particularly regarding reproductive function (Domar et al., 1990).

When you experience psychological stress, your brain triggers a response called the hypothalamic-pituitary-adrenal (HPA) axis, which has previously been discussed in this book. This results in signals being sent that instruct the adrenal glands to produce stress hormones, like cortisol. While this response is helpful when there is a real threat to your life, prolonged or chronic activation from psychological stressors is not helpful.

Chronic stress poses significant risks, as it can interfere with essential reproductive processes such as ovulation, sperm production, and implantation. Research supports, elevated levels of stress hormones can disrupt the secretion of reproductive hormones, resulting in irregular menstrual cycles for women and diminished fertility for men. The cumulative effects of ongoing stress can therefore notably reduce the likelihood of conception, highlighting the importance of managing stress for individuals aiming to conceive.

Evidence also suggests that high levels of psychological stress can adversely affect the success rates of fertility treatments, (Domar et.el.,2011) indicating the necessity of incorporating mental health support within reproductive healthcare. Rotimi and Singh (2024) contend that lifestyle stressors such as smoking, alcohol and lack of exercise also play a critical role in reproductive health, therefore, it is crucial to understand the complex interplay between physical and emotional stress and reproductive health to develop comprehensive strategies that promote fertility and enhance overall well-being.

Hypnotherapy can facilitate deep relaxation and stress reduction, providing a holistic means to rebalance the individual. As we know, unlike traditional talk therapies, hypnotherapy operates at a subconscious level, addressing entrenched beliefs and emotional blockages that often lie hidden beneath the surface. By targeting these underlying issues, hypnotherapy assists individuals in achieving a state of emotional and physical alignment conducive to conception.

Sessions focused on infertility are highly personalised, catering to the unique emotional landscapes and needs of individuals or couples. Stress reduction serves as the cornerstone of this approach, with sessions typically beginning with progressive relaxation techniques that guide clients into a state of deep physical and mental calm. This relaxation alleviates the physiological effects of stress, creating an environment where the subconscious mind is more receptive to positive suggestions due to the physiological changes that happen in the brain as we read about in chapter 6. *The Brain in Trance: The Neuroscience of Hypnotherapy.*

Many individuals grappling with infertility carry deep-seated fears and guilt, often expressing thoughts such as, "My body is broken," "I will never be a parent," or "It's my fault." In my many years of working with this group, I can assure you that it is seldom the fault of any one person, even when it may appear so to the outside world. Holding on to blame is certainly unhelpful, and if our clients are doing so, we must assist them in reframing these thoughts and releasing the associated judgement. Hypnotherapy aims to identify and reshape these negative beliefs, transforming, for instance, the thought "My body is broken" into "In the past, I have struggled, but my body knows how to heal, and I am open to new possibilities."

Clients are equipped with tools to recognise the thoughts leading them to suboptimal outcomes and are taught mindful processes of non-judgement that allow such thoughts to pass without criticism. Additionally, visualisation plays a significant role in the process. Clients are guided to envision their bodies functioning optimally, picturing their reproductive organs as healthy and receptive, while also imagining the joy of holding their baby. These visualisations help align the subconscious mind with the desired outcome, reinforcing hope and motivation.

However, it can be challenging to ask an infertile client to imagine achieving success. For many, this can lead to feelings of failure, as IVF and other infertility treatments often have limited success rates, and outcomes are not always positive. Thus, this process must be approached with understanding, compassion, and in consultation with the client. I have found it helpful to encourage clients to visualise the next step in their journey, rather than focusing on the final destination. For example, if they are undergoing IVF and preparing for egg collection, I guide them to imagine their eggs maturing. If it is after an embryo transfer, I encourage them to visualise a fertile endometrial lining ready to receive an embryo and to picture the embryo implanting.

This imagery does not need to be physiologically accurate, as long as the client can develop a clear sense of it for themselves. Often, I use a Goldilocks metaphor for embryo implantation, where the embryo finds the part of the uterine lining that is "just right" and settles in for a beautiful rest, pulling up the covers as it comfortably positions itself.

As for all client groups hypnotherapy provides a safe space to address emotional blockages caused by past traumas, unresolved grief, or relationship conflicts that can, in this client group, hinder conception. Techniques such as age regression enable clients to revisit and heal from past experiences that may be contributing to their current struggles.

Research has shown the efficacy of hypnotherapy as a complementary treatment for infertility. A study by Levitas et al. (2006) demonstrated that using hypnosis during embryo transfer in IVF significantly increased pregnancy rates. Similarly, Domar et al. (2011) found that psychological interventions, including hypnotherapy, led to higher conception rates and reduced stress levels in women undergoing fertility treatments. While more extensive studies are necessary, these findings are not surprising to hypnotherapists working in this area, and they underscore the potential of hypnotherapy to improve both emotional well-being and physiological outcomes.

I believe that hypnotherapy is perfectly poised to work side by side with assisted reproductive technologies, creating a dynamic synergistic interplay where the combination of both practices amplifies their individual strengths. Together forming a powerful alliance, producing effects that are greater than the sum of their individual parts, strengthening the journey towards conception with a harmonious blend of psychological and physiological support.

This holistic approach to fertility, particularly when combined with medical interventions, proper nutrition, and lifestyle adjustments, can significantly enhance overall well-being. Incorporating mindfulness practices alongside hypnotherapy further supports stress reduction, while dietary changes and moderate exercise contribute to improved reproductive health. Working collaboratively with medical professionals can ensure that clients receive comprehensive care tailored to their individual needs.

Infertility, therefore, is not just a physical condition; it is a deeply emotional and psychological interplay and hypnotherapy can offer a compassionate, non-invasive approach to addressing the psychological and emotional dimensions of fertility challenges. By fostering a state of empowered calm, reframing limiting beliefs, and empowering individuals to safely visualise success one step at a time, hypnotherapy provides a pathway toward healing and hope.

As the field of hypnotherapy continues to evolve, its integration into fertility care holds immense potential. By addressing mind-body potential, we can help individuals move closer to their dream of parenthood, one peaceful, transformative session at a time.

Case Study: Julie's Journey Through Hypnotherapy for Infertility

Julie is a 34-year-old woman who has been struggling with infertility for 18 months, having been unable to conceive despite regular unprotected intercourse. Alongside her fertility challenges, she is also caring for her ailing mother-in-law while managing a full-time job. This combination of responsibilities has left Julie feeling exhausted, overwhelmed and anxious. She experiences constant worry about her inability to conceive, intensifying her feelings of guilt and fear of not meeting both her and her partner's dreams of becoming parents. She states she has trouble sleeping at night due to the intrusive thoughts.

During Julie's initial session, she expressed deep frustration stemming from her infertility journey and the emotional toll it has taken on her. She mentioned the monthly disappointment each time her period arrived, combined with feelings of inadequacy, often thinking, "Am I broken?" or "What's wrong with me?" These thoughts were often compounded by her caregiving responsibilities and job stress. Julie felt there was no time for herself. Together, we established the goals for her therapy: to alleviate her anxiety, manage her responsibilities and find time for herself, reduce her stress by learning helpful techniques she could implement at home, enhance her emotional resilience, and foster a positive mindset towards conception.

Hypnotherapy Sessions:

Over the course of several sessions, the following techniques were employed to address Julie's infertility concerns:

Deep Relaxation Techniques

Each session began with progressive relaxation exercises, helping Julie create a calm mental state. This relaxation not only alleviated her immediate anxiety but also allowed her to let go of worries about her fertility and embrace positive thoughts and affirmations.

Reframing Negative Beliefs

Julie was asked to observe and challenge her negative self-talk. One important example was to change her focus from infertility to fertility. Statements such as "I'm infertile" became "I'm strengthening my fertility" or "my infertility journey" became "my fertility journey". Julie also often carried the belief that she was somehow personally responsible for failing in her journey to conceive. Through guided hypnotherapy, we worked to reframe these negative self-perceptions. We transformed her thoughts of "I can't get pregnant" into "My body is capable and knows exactly what to do", "my body knows how to heal and restore" and "I am open to normal, healthy outcomes." This shift empowered her to approach her fertility journey with hope rather than despair.

Visualisation

We employed visualisation techniques, guiding Julie to imagine her body functioning optimally for conception. She envisioned healthy reproductive organs welcoming a fertilised embryo, picturing herself feeling joy and love as she embraced her future child. This positive imagery helped align her subconscious mind with her goal of conception.

Addressing Anxiety Triggers

We explored the specific situations that heightened Julie's anxiety about infertility. In several sessions, we used age regression techniques to delve into her past experiences and insecurities that contributed to her present feelings of unworthiness. This exploration allowed Julie to understand and release deep-seated fears, enabling her to move forward with greater confidence.

Mindfulness Practice

To further support her emotional well-being, we incorporated mindfulness techniques. Julie learned to observe her anxious thoughts without judgement, allowing them to pass without impacting her sense of self-worth. She allowed herself to be here and now in the present moment, not back in the past ruminating over the things she could not change, and not out in the future imagining her worst scenario. This practice helped her cultivate a more positive mindset during her fertility journey.

Breath Techniques

Breathing techniques were employed and practised daily, alongside a recorded progressive muscle relaxation that Julie listened to twice a day. This combination encouraged her nervous system to connect with parasympathetic functioning and initiated the process of rewiring her brain for greater calmness and positivity through a process of neural rewiring.

Self-Care

The importance of self-care was emphasised as Julie recognised that she could not pour from an empty cup; she needed to replenish, restore, and recuperate to care for others effectively.

The Power of Repetition

This concept was reinforced as paramount. Julie was instructed to notice any persistent and unhelpful thoughts without judgement, allowing them to float away as easily as they had appeared. She learned that the less attention she gave these thoughts, the less frequently they would arise. This realisation became a powerful affirmation of her ability to direct her own change.

After a series of six sessions, Julie reported significant improvements in her anxiety levels and overall emotional well-being. She expressed feeling more in control of her thoughts regarding her infertility, experiencing fewer feelings of despair. Julie's sleep improved, and she found herself able to concentrate better at work. With a newfound ability to approach her fertility journey with optimism, she began to engage more meaningfully with her partner, focusing on the love and support they shared rather than solely on the goal of conception.

Julie developed a deeper understanding of the importance of self-care and started incorporating short mindfulness practices into her daily routine. By the end of our sessions, she felt empowered to embrace her journey towards motherhood with confidence, viewing it as a shared experience with her partner rather than a burden she carried alone.

Six months later Julie reported that she was 10 weeks pregnant with their first child. She was excited for the future and expressed she would continue her daily practices throughout the pregnancy.

In conclusion, this case study highlights how hypnotherapy can support individuals like Julie, who face the complex challenges of infertility. By addressing the emotional and psychological factors contributing to her anxiety, hypnotherapy fostered resilience and offered a holistic approach to enhance her journey toward conception.

Chapter Twenty-Three

HYPNOTHERAPY AS A SUPPORTIVE APPROACH FOR AUTOIMMUNE DISORDERS

Autoimmune disorders arise when the immune system mistakenly identifies the body's own tissues as foreign invaders. This misconception often results in chronic inflammation, pain, and a range of debilitating symptoms. Conditions such as rheumatoid arthritis, psoriatic arthritis, lupus, type 1 diabetes, multiple sclerosis and Hashimoto's thyroiditis to name but a few disorders, affect millions worldwide. These stem from a complex interplay of genetic, environmental, and psychological factors (Davidson & Diamond, 2001). While conventional treatments, including immunosuppressive drugs and anti-inflammatory medications, are often essential, it is equally important to address the psychological and emotional components of these conditions.

Hypnotherapy is a valuable complementary mind-body approach that can assist patients in managing autoimmune disorders by enhancing their quality of life, reducing stress, and fostering a greater sense of control over their symptoms. The connection between chronic stress and autoimmune disorders is well documented, with unresolved emotional trauma further exacerbating these conditions by dysregulating the immune system. Once again we see the hypothalamic-pituitary-adrenal (HPA) axis, which regulates stress responses, is often over-activated in individuals with chronic illnesses. Prolonged activation of the HPA axis can lead to a shift in immune regulation from anti-inflammatory to pro-inflammatory, ultimately promoting chronic inflammation and the release of pro-inflammatory cytokines, worsening autoimmune conditions. (Hou & Li, 2014).

As we have discussed many times previously in this book, stress is a factor in so many conditions and hypnotherapy can play a crucial role in calming the HPA axis and reducing stress levels. By addressing subconscious thought patterns and emotional responses that may contribute to illness, hypnotherapy can help to foster a deep sense of calm and promotes a positive healing internal environment and mindset through cognitive restructuring and supportive mental imagery. This process activates the body's natural healing mechanisms, paving the way for a transition from chronic inflammation to a state of healing and balance, essential for individuals with autoimmune disorders.

Achieving deep states of relaxation can initiate various physiological responses: decreasing the production of stress hormones like cortisol and adrenaline, chronic over-activation of which is known to exacerbate inflammation, and encourages positive mental imagery, allowing patients to visualise their bodies in a state of health and wellness. This enhances emotional resilience and promotes effective coping strategies. Research indicates that this mind-body connection can significantly bolster immune responses, aiding in symptom management and influencing disease progression (Henney & Hackett, 2025).

As highlighted throughout this book, addressing fundamental underlying factors affecting client's general health is imperative. Stress often being a significant contributor must be addressed. When the body experiences stress, it activates the fight-or-flight response, a survival mechanism discussed previously. This response triggers the sympathetic nervous system, leading to the release of stress hormones like adrenaline and cortisol. Although beneficial in acute situations by increasing heart rate, blood pressure, and energy supply to muscles, chronic stress can have detrimental effects on the body's capacity to heal (Sapolsky, 2004).

In prolonged stress, the body prioritises immediate survival over healing and recovery. During this state, the immune system becomes suppressed as resources are redirected to manage the perceived threat (McEwen, 2007). Consequently, the body struggles to combat diseases and repair itself, leading to increased inflammation, a common factor in many health issues, including autoimmune conditions. Chronic activation of the sympathetic nervous system can also disrupt digestion, increase muscle tension, and cause fatigue, further hindering the body's natural healing processes.

Techniques that activate the parasympathetic nervous system, including cognitive awareness tools, hypnotic relaxation practices, daily recorded guided hypnotic sessions, and breathing exercises focused on parasympathetic nervous system activation, can counteract the stress response. By promoting a state of calm, these strategies facilitate recovery and restore the body's balance, allowing for more efficient healing.

Hypnotherapy offers a range of effective tools and applications to support clients dealing with autoimmune conditions, which when frequently accompanied by heightened states of stress and tension, may trigger painful flare-ups. Therefore, a longer induction is often beneficial for these clients. Hypnotherapy sessions may typically begin with progressive muscle relaxation combined with therapeutic suggestions and guided imagery directed toward a softening, releasing and letting go, allowing clients to enter a state of deep physical and mental calm. This relaxation promotes stress reduction and can activate a healing environment within the body enhancing the potential for recovery. Effective examples of suggestions whilst in the hypnotic state may be "*As you enter this beautiful state of deepest relaxation your body has nothing else to do but function perfectly and perfectly function.*" Or "*You have now entered the state beneath the level of conscious aware-*

ness where true healing happens... easily and effortlessly... when there is nothing else to do".

Clients are guided to visualise their immune systems functioning optimally and importantly, normally, with no requirement for a precise physiological understanding of their body's complex processes. It is sufficient to know and believe that just as their body knew how to create a functioning healthy immune system, it knows how to heal that same system. Even though the client may not know how to do this consciously, they *do* know beneath the level of conscious awareness. I would offer a suggestion such as "and even though you may not know how to heal your immune system, consciously, you can be reassured to remember that the same intelligence that created it in the first place, does know, so you don't need to know consciously." Or "Your subconscious mind knows what your conscious mind does not need to know so you can just relax and let your body find balance again, just like before."

Clients are encouraged to create images that resonate personally with them. For instance, some clients envision their immune systems as an army of tiny blueberry warriors bravely engaging in battle against foreign invaders, whilst easily sparing normal healthy cells and tissues, a concept inspired by a popular advertisement for probiotic gut health. Others may picture their immune cells as little Pac-Men, energetically gobbling up only harmful entities and resting when the job is done. Some may imagine their healthy tissues in a team colour whilst the invaders are in another colour, easily distinguishable to the immune system so that friendly fire is always avoided during battle. Additionally, I have had children imagine their immune systems as purple flying dragons, which they could ride into battle, emerging victorious over adversaries. There is no right or wrong representation; for musically inclined clients, their immune cells might be envisioned as a harmonious orchestra, working in perfect balance. These vivid images support the subconscious mind in fostering healing and reprogramming more positive thought patterns.

Chronic illness in the form of autoimmune disorders often lead to negative self-perceptions, such as "My body has failed me" or "I have no control over my health." Hypnotherapy can help clients identify and reframe these beliefs, replacing them with empowering affirmations like "My body is resilient and knows how to heal", "My body has healed many times in the past" or "I am an active participant in my health journey." It is essential for us to listen closely to our clients' language, paying attention to the words they use that may be self-limiting. We should note how often they employ terms like "should," "can't," "always," and "never," and explore the underlying statements connected to them, as these reveal their self-narrative. As we know well by now, the subconscious mind will respond to our every thought and molecules of emotion stem from our thoughts, words and beliefs. Therefore, once again our clients must be careful with the labels they choose to hold. Even subtle changes to the client's narrative such as referring to 'the condition' instead of 'my autoimmune condition' can make a difference.

Recognising limiting beliefs is crucial, as they generally operate at a subconscious level and manifest as self-fulfilling prophecies that will hinder progress. By bringing these statements into conscious awareness, we empower our clients to evaluate their validity, allowing them to decide if these beliefs serve their well-being and determine the actions they choose to take moving forward.

The existence of underlying emotional trauma will also need to be identified, as unresolved emotional trauma may also contribute to the exacerbation of autoimmune symptoms. Techniques such as age regression, described in earlier chapters, can allow clients to safely revisit and release past traumas that may be influencing their current health. This emotional release can profoundly impact physical symptoms and overall well-being.

CASE STUDY: EMILY'S JOURNEY WITH MULTIPLE SCLEROSIS

Emily, a 38-year-old graphic designer, was diagnosed with multiple sclerosis (MS) five years prior. The diagnosis, characterised by unpredictable flare-ups and debilitating fatigue, profoundly impacted her daily life, relationships, and sense of self. She suffered greatly from fatigue, poor sleep, relationship decline. Because of her self-identity as a person with a degenerative disease, she became increasingly future focused, often in the most catastrophic ways. This habit of taking herself out to the future directly to her worst scenarios was preventing her from living in the present moment and adding to her feelings of overwhelm. Despite following a conventional medical treatment plan, she struggled with anxiety over her symptoms and the unpredictability of her condition, which often led to feelings of hopelessness and frustration.

Before going further, let's understand exactly what MS is. In many ways MS is like a case of mistaken identity within the body. The immune system, which is usually our loyal guard dog, trained to protect us from outside invaders, suddenly becomes confused. Instead of defending us, it turns inward, mistaking the body's own tissues for an enemy. In MS, the target of this misplaced attack is the myelin sheath, the soft insulating layer that wraps around our nerve fibres in the brain and spinal cord.

You might think of myelin as the plastic coating around an electrical wire. It keeps the current flowing cleanly and efficiently, ensuring the message gets from one end to the other without interference. When the immune system chews away at this protective layer the messages between the brain and the body stutter, slow down, or sometimes never arrive at all. It's a bit like static crackling over a phone line, or a frayed wire that flickers unpredictably.

This confusion begins when certain immune cells, especially T-cells, slip through the brain's natural security gate, the blood–brain barrier. Once inside, they send out distress calls, drawing in other immune cells, including B-cells, to join the mistaken battle. Together, they create inflammation, strip away myelin, and often leave behind hardened scars, known as plaques. These plaques act like potholes on a road interrupting the smooth passage of signals and leaving the nervous system struggling to keep communication flowing.

For those living with MS, the result can be a patchwork of experiences: blurred vision one day, a heavy fatigue the next. Balance and movement can falter on some occasions while thoughts or memories can feel out of reach at other times. The course of the condition is thus, unpredictable. Symptoms may ease for a while and then suddenly creep forward.

At its heart, MS is the story of an immune system that has lost its way: a protector turned aggressor, unsettling the harmony of the body's most delicate communication network.

In search of relief and empowerment in managing her condition, Emily sought out an alternative approach and turned to hypnotherapy. During her initial consultation, she expressed concerns about her ongoing fatigue and troubled sleep patterns, alongside the emotional burden stemming from her diagnosis.

As with so many of our clients who present into the consulting room, Emily was naturally very problem focused. Each day she would go in search of the symptoms of her disease, noticing the intensity and looking for signs of them worsening and as expected, just like shining a torch into the darkness, she was able to find what she was looking for.

From the outside looking in, It became evident that the principle of "what we focus on, we strengthen," was at play here (Kabat-Zinn, 1990). By concentrating on the constructive aspects of her journey, and the things she was able to control, we aimed to shine that light in a different direction and enhance her resilience.

The first step in this process was to clearly define the problems she was encountering and how they were impacting her life. From here we were able to formulate a personalised Hypnotherapy plan designed to find solutions to these problems that would assist Emily to reduce stress and anxiety, manage symptoms, and cultivate a renewed sense of hope for the future.

In the initial sessions, as has been well discussed in previous chapters, I educated Emily about the power and potential of the mind and body to work together in synergistically dynamic ways. The importance of noting her self-talk, expectations and focus of attention were all discussed within the framework of the physiology of the body and the predictable outcomes such as; what you think you will feel, and what you focus on becomes magnified. As with all my clients this pre-talk becomes the foundation for creating an empowered state on which to build successful change.

Cognitive awareness and reframing exercises were introduced, and Emily learned how to notice and challenge negative beliefs about her condition, such as "I am losing control of my body." She was taught to notice these thoughts and to release them without judgement. Judgement, as we know, would only give them even more attention and strength, which was definitely not the desired outcome. Instead, we worked together to replace such thoughts with Emily's own solution focused statements such as, "I am resilient, and my body is strong." She was asked to embody the statement, really connecting to the feeling of her solution state, imagining herself healthy and strong, importantly 'in this moment'. Embodying her goal state, in 'the now', allows her subconscious mind to respond to her thoughts and feelings, as if they are real and true in this moment, and thus, the chemistry of her goal state is created.

A clear vision of her realistic goal was identified, which included slowing the progression of her disease by reducing stress and therefore creating an optimal internal environment for healing, effectively managing and minimising her associated physical and psychological symptoms, and creating an empowered expectancy of hope for her future. A respectful appreciation of the intricate interplay between the mind and body was fostered. Emily understood that she was to play an active part in this process, and her focus of attention and heightened awareness of how to strengthen her outcomes by embodying a healthy mindset were imperative.

One key aspect of our hypnotic work involved visualisation techniques, where Emily imagined her body surrounded by a warm, healing light. This light symbolised both comfort and strength, representing her body's innate ability to heal itself. Times when her body had been able to do just that, in the past, were identified and became the basis for therapeutic suggestions whilst in trance. She had healed from coughs, colds, viruses, scrapes, cuts and even a broken leg in the past. Her body already knew how to heal and return to optimal health. She was directed to look for positive changes and notice them all.

Importantly she was instructed that the work she did between sessions was just as important as the work we were doing in session, in fact even more. This had a two-fold intention. To empower Emily to know that she was driving her own outcomes, not me, and to introduce the power of repetition for creation change as previously described in chapter nine. The more she stepped away from stress by using the self-hypnotic progressive muscle relaxation and visualisations, the faster she began seeing positive results.

As Emily continued her hypnotherapy sessions, and her daily cognitive and self-hypnotic practices, she reported gradual but noticeable improvements. The more improvements she noticed the more she was inspired to do the homework tasks, which were now becoming her daily self-care practices. She experienced less anxiety about her condition, and more positive hope for the future. This allowed her to participate in and manage the requirements of daily life more effectively.

The emotional toll MS had taken on Emily was explored through regression where the feeling she had connected to, took her all the way back to early childhood past trauma. She recounted a challenging period from her childhood involving bullying, which had led to lingering feelings of anxiety and inadequacy. We explored this and how this may have contributed to her tendency toward anxiety throughout life, anxiety that had now been exacerbated by her current diagnosis. Through this exploration, Emily was able to make significant connections between her childhood experiences and her current fears surrounding her illness. With further exploration she was able to release the negative feelings associated with those memories, allowing her to cultivate a greater sense of self-worth and autonomy. The realisation that her value was not defined by others' opinions or actions and not by her current health condition led to a deeper understanding that was truly liberating for her.

As she entered the clinic on session six, approximately two months after commencing therapy, she stated she felt she had returned to the land of the living and had a strong feeling of hope that there was a future for her, and she would be the one to create it. Also stating that this diagnosis was not going to define her. Her sleep had improved as she utilised the relaxation and cognitive techniques learned in sessions to quiet her mind at night. She reported this newfound ability to relax, sleep well and control her thoughts had significantly enhanced her personal relationships and her overall quality of life.

Emily now feels empowered and more in control of her life. She has developed effective coping strategies to manage her symptoms and anxiety. The progress she has made is remarkable; she has embraced her diagnosis rather than resisting it and allowing it to define her. Emily's case illustrates the potential of hypnotherapy as a valuable tool in the holistic treatment of autoimmune disorders, demonstrating the profound impact it can have on both physical symptoms and emotional resilience. Her journey with multiple sclerosis continues, but she faces it with newfound confidence, strength, and a sense of hope for the future.

Studies on the effects of hypnotherapy on stress reduction also highlight its potential to positively influence the immune system. A review by Gruzelier (2002) demonstrated that hypnosis can alleviate stress-induced immune dysregulation, paving the way for improved symptom management in autoimmune disorders. Research has increasingly demonstrated the benefits of hypnotherapy for managing autoimmune disorders, including multiple sclerosis (MS). A systematic review and meta-analysis by Thompson et al. (2019) concluded that hypnotherapy effectively reduces pain perception and anxiety, both of which are known triggers for exacerbations in autoimmune disorders. By facilitating relaxation and altering the perception of pain, hypnotherapy serves as a complementary approach that empowers patients to better manage their symptoms and fosters a greater sense of control over their health journey. These findings underscore the potential of hypnotherapy as a valuable tool in holistic treatment strategies for individuals living with autoimmune disorders such as MS.

What we see in the clinic is that hypnotherapy can be very effective when integrated into a holistic treatment plan, which may include medical interventions, dietary changes, exercise, and stress-management techniques like cognitive processes, self-hypnotic visualisations, meditation, breathwork, or mindfulness. Autoimmune disorders present a complex challenge that affects both the body and mind. Hypnotherapy offers a compassionate, non-invasive approach to managing these conditions by addressing the psychological and emotional factors that can exacerbate symptoms.

This combination allowed Emily to address the emotional and psychological aspects of her illness, empowering her to reclaim her sense of self and significantly improve her quality of life. By fostering deep relaxation, reframing limiting beliefs, and promoting emotional healing, hypnotherapy enables individuals like Emily to take an active role in their health journey. It significantly enhances health outcomes and serves as a powerful complement to medical treatments, offering hope and relief to those living with autoimmune disorders.

Chapter Twenty-Four

HYPNOTHERAPY IN THE MANAGEMENT OF INFLAMMATION AND ARTHRITIS

The principles of hypnotherapy are particularly relevant within the context of chronic conditions such as generalised inflammation or arthritis. As stated by the ancient philosopher Hippocrates, “It is more important to know what sort of person has a disease than to know what sort of disease a person has.” This wisdom highlights the importance of holistic treatment approaches, especially for individuals suffering from inflammatory conditions.

So why do we become inflamed? Inflammation serves as the body's natural defence mechanism. It acts as an alarm system whose job it is to respond to injury or infection. In its acute form, it is beneficial, bringing blood, nutrients, and immune cells to the affected area to promote healing. However, as we saw in the previous chapter, when this alarm continues to sound without a real threat, the body begins to suffer.

Chronic inflammation can manifest as fatigue, joint pain and digestive issues which can strip individuals of their vitality and zest for life (Schmidt et al., 2023). This relentless condition can be metaphorically likened to a car engine that overheats, with warning lights signifying an underlying issue that, if neglected, could lead to catastrophic failure.

Akin to a bushfire raging out of control, ongoing chronic inflammation can lead to various health conditions, including cardiovascular disease, diabetes, rheumatoid arthritis, certain cancers and autoimmune disorders. In today's fast-paced world, the delicate balance of the natural inflammatory process is easily disrupted, unleashing a cascade of destructive consequences.

Hypnosis serves as a unique restorative process for individuals grappling with chronic inflammation. By fostering a state of focused awareness and deep relaxation, hypnosis allows patients to access their subconscious minds, confronting sources of discomfort and eliciting profound healing responses. This therapeutic technique not only alleviates pain but also enhances emotional well-being, addressing the psychological components of inflammation (Brown et al., 2017).

Research supports the efficacy of hypnosis in significantly reducing inflammation-related symptoms. Much study has been done looking at inflammatory bowel disease that has supported that participants with IBS experienced substantial decreases in disease activity following multiple hypnosis sessions. Results indicated not only physical improvements but also notable enhancements in emotional health, showcasing the dual benefits of this therapeutic approach.

The therapeutic benefits of hypnosis stem from its capacity to modulate the body's stress response. Again, we see our nemesis, chronic stress, being a key contributor to inflammation, elevating cortisol levels that exacerbate inflammatory conditions.

As we have observed in previous chapters, by promoting relaxation and reducing stress, hypnosis helps lower cortisol levels, paving the way for repair and recovery. Hypnosis also enhances the body's innate healing capabilities. Utilising visualisation techniques, individuals mentally engage with their condition, promoting a sense of control and empowerment in the face of chronic pain, ultimately leading to actual physiological changes. Further to this, hypnotherapy's relevance to arthritis lies in its ability to modify pain perception and reduce emotional distress associated with chronic pain. Patients with rheumatoid arthritis who utilised hypnotherapy have reported marked reductions in pain and improvements in joint function, alongside enhanced emotional resilience.

In summary, practical applications of hypnotherapy in the management of inflammation and arthritis involve several key approaches. Firstly, pain relief can be achieved through techniques like guided imagery, which help patients visualise their pain diminishing, effectively decreasing the perception of discomfort. On a physiological level, when the brain shifts into a calmer state, it releases natural chemicals like endorphins which act like the body's natural painkillers, easing discomfort and calming inflammation.

Suggestions that illuminate research based physiological changes, such as this, that occur in the state of hypnosis can be very powerful convincers that can assist in shifting our client's expectancy toward successful outcomes. Pathways that quieten the nervous system are also activated in the hypnotic state. These changes not only reduce the perception of pain but also help lower the body's inflammatory response. Regular hypnotherapy sessions also facilitate stress reduction by cultivating deep relaxation, thereby lowering stress levels that contribute to inflammation and pain relief.

Hypnotherapy also encourages behavioural change by fostering motivation for healthier lifestyle choices, such as increased physical activity and improved nutrition, which promote active self-care practices. Additionally, it can offer emotional healing by providing a safe space for individuals to explore their feelings of frustration and despair. This also fosters resilience in the face of chronic pain. Therefore, by teaching our clients to influence their pain experience in positive ways, hypnotherapy encourages a sense of empowerment and control, significantly enhancing the emotional and physical well-being of our clients.

CASE STUDY: JILLIAN'S JOURNEY TO HEALING

One compelling example of the power of hypnotherapy is Jillian, a 63-year-old retired teacher who had been living with rheumatoid arthritis for over a decade. Her days were often filled with chronic pain, joint stiffness, and fatigue. Despite medication and physical therapy, periods of stress frequently triggered symptom flare-ups, leaving her feeling powerless and disconnected from her body.

In search of a complementary approach to her treatment plan, Jillian turned to hypnotherapy. During her initial consultation, she shared her struggles with stress and expressed feelings of frustration over her perceived lack of control. Together, we developed a personalised hypnotherapy plan aimed at reducing stress, managing pain, and fostering a sense of self-empowerment.

In the first few sessions, we focused on deep relaxation and pain management. We examined her self-talk, including the unhelpful statements she told herself, her expectations, and her ability to recognise these thoughts to create a shift in her mindset. Breath-work was an integral part of the therapeutic direction to assist her in managing the levels of stress she encountered daily. During these initial sessions, we also worked on developing a sense of hopefulness and an expectancy of change. Cognitive techniques were employed to explore her body's responses to her thought patterns, which reinforced her ability to step out of stress just as swiftly as she had stepped into it.

Jillian was guided into a state of calm and taught to visualise her joints bathed in soothing, healing light. She reported that these visualisations not only eased her pain but also improved her sleep quality. Through a self-hypnotic breath technique that she learned to enter at will, her body was able to quickly enter a state of deep calm in which optimal functioning and healing was possible. She was instructed to continue practising this between sessions.

As the therapy progressed, we addressed Jillian's previous feelings of helplessness. Through positive suggestion and visualisation, she was able to shift her mindset, replacing despairing thoughts such as “I can’t do this anymore” with affirmations like “I am strong, and my body is working with me.”

During a session of regression, we explored past emotional traumas that may have contributed to her current physical condition. Jillian revealed that she had experienced a significant loss in her early forties: the miscarriage of a hard-fought pregnancy after a long battle with infertility, a loss she had never fully processed. Through gentle exploration, she was able to forgive herself and finally release the long-held guilt stemming from a belief that she bore some responsibility for the loss of her baby.

The persistent notion that “her body had failed her” and was “broken” had seemingly contributed to the persistence of the arthritis which proved her underlying belief, that her body was broken and had failed her, again. Through a dissociation technique, where she was able to observe another woman in exactly the same situation and offer that woman love and compassion for her loss, Jillian was able to offer herself the same compassion as she had given to the other woman. She confronted and released the unresolved grief that she believed had been weighing her down both emotionally and physically, entering a state of self-acceptance and self-love. This combined with the understanding that it was never her fault led to a significant abreaction, which allowed Jillian to finally express her sorrow for the mother she was not to become and for her unborn child.

Importantly, an abreaction should not be feared. Jillian was permitted to experience her emotions for as long as she needed, after I first ensured it was safe for her to do so. She sobbed uncontrollably for a full ten minutes before the tears slowed, and she took a long, slow deep breath, letting it all go. When she emerged from the trance, she thanked me for allowing her to experience that release; she had not realised the extent to which she had held onto the misplaced guilt from that time.

Ongoing hypnotherapy sessions saw a reduction in Jillian’s arthritic symptoms. She reported a substantial reduction in her flare-ups, and while she still experienced occasional pain, she felt better equipped to manage her condition both physically and emotionally. Months later she was able to reduce her anti-inflammatory medication with the approval of her treating physician. Her improved outlook on life and ability to cope enhanced her personal relationships and overall quality of life, demonstrating the transformative potential of integrating hypnotherapy into her treatment.

Importantly Jillian continued doing all of her self-care techniques, monitoring her self-talk, interrupting unhelpful cognitions and practiced daily breath work and short guided visualisation and hypnotic meditations.

Research corroborates the efficacy of hypnotherapy as a complementary approach for managing chronic illnesses, including autoimmune disorders. For example, a study by Gay et al. (2012) found that hypnosis significantly reduced pain and improved quality of life in patients with rheumatoid arthritis. Similarly, Jensen et al. (2009) reported that hypnosis effectively decreased chronic pain intensity and enhanced emotional well-being in individuals with autoimmune conditions, such as arthritis. Both provide compelling evidence supporting the use of hypnotherapy for such conditions.

We now see more frequently that hypnosis is emerging as a powerful ally in managing chronic inflammation. By enhancing relaxation, improving pain perception, and addressing the emotional causes of chronic pain, this therapeutic technique offers a comprehensive approach to healing for our clients. As illustrated through the stories of individuals such as Jillian, hypnotherapy not only has the potential to transform physical health outcomes but also has the ability to cultivate emotional resilience.

What we therefore observe in our clients is an ability to become empowered to manage the complexities of their own conditions using practical self-help hypnotherapeutic tools. This fosters within our clients a hope for the future and cultivates a genuine sense of expectancy that change is not only possible, but also inevitable, as they learn how to effectively integrate the potential of the body and mind to achieve recovery.

> To quote Candice Pert, PhD, from an excerpt from "Your Body is Your Subconscious Mind": "*Your body is the outward manifestation of your mind.*"

Therefore, let us all harness the power of our thoughts and emotions to shape our realities, empowering ourselves to take charge of our health and transform the trajectory of our lives.

Chapter Twenty-Five

HYPNOTHERAPY FOR POST TRAUMATIC STRESS DISORDER (PTSD): RECLAIMING CONTROL.

Post-Traumatic Stress Disorder (PTSD) is a debilitating condition that leaves individuals feeling trapped in an endless loop of relived trauma. Characterised by intrusive memories, hypervigilance, emotional numbing, and avoidance behaviours, PTSD disrupts the lives of those who endure it, often eroding their sense of safety and control. Hypnotherapy offers a transformative approach to healing PTSD by interrupting and redirecting the subconscious mind's unhelpful narratives.

As a clinical hypnotherapist and counsellor, I've observed the profound changes hypnotherapy can bring to individuals with PTSD. By safely accessing the subconscious mind, where traumatic memories reside, hypnotherapy can allow clients to reframe their experiences and rewrite the narratives connected to them, diminishing emotional triggers and empowering them to move forward with a hopeful expectancy that life can be different.

One of the main concerns with working in this area is that the person may be re-traumatised, and this we need to avoid at all costs. Therefore, as with all disorders, we need to have a good understanding of it in order to work effectively with it. I again caution here that if you are not confident and competent to work in this area, you really should not.

PTSD is a natural response to an overwhelming event that exceeds the person's capacity to cope. Whether precipitated by war, abuse, accidents, natural disasters, or other life-threatening experiences, the trauma becomes embedded in the subconscious mind, influencing thoughts, behaviours, and physiological responses.

We must remember here that it is the bodies prime function to protect you. Due to this survival instinct, the perceived threat is stored in an area of the brain, where it can immediately be reactivated, unfortunately this often occurs inappropriately. When faced with reminders of the trauma, the brain's survival mechanisms can trigger a fight-or-flight response, even when the individual is no longer in danger. Over time, this heightened state of arousal can lead to chronic stress, anxiety, depression, and various physical health issues (Yehuda et al., 2015).

Hypnotherapy can be useful in these instances by accessing the subconscious mind, where memories and emotions associated with trauma are stored. This allows the hypnotherapist to help clients process these memories in a safe and controlled manner.

In my practise I incorporate a compassionate, client-centred approach to hypnotherapy for PTSD, gently guiding and supporting clients as they access their inner resilience and ability to rewrite the problematic subconscious narratives that have been holding them back.

With this safe approach, I've seen clients transition from feeling broken by their trauma to recognising their strength to overcome it. It is important to understand that hypnotherapy can't erase the past, but it can change the way our clients perceive the past and therefore, how the past affects the present. Hypnotherapy for PTSD is all about supporting our clients to free themselves from the old version of the past so that they can move forward.

So how do we safely work with this client group and what are some of the important things to bear in mind when working with PTSD? First and foremost, establishing a safe environment for this client group must be our highest priority. The essence of effective therapy hinges on our ability to build trust and rapport and to cultivate a safe comfortable therapeutic environment where our client feels able to explore the underlying causative issues. This is essential for those who have been grappling with the elusive nature of distress and anxiety that often accompanies PTSD which can manifest in a myriad of symptoms, each intricately woven into the fabric of an individual's psyche.

Those afflicted may find themselves haunted by intrusive memories, reliving their trauma through harrowing flashbacks or restless nights plagued by nightmares. In their quest for relief, many adopt avoidance strategies, avoiding reminders of the past, be it in the form of familiar places, people, or activities that once brought joy. The emotional toll of PTSD often runs deeper than what we see on the surface; individuals may grapple with persistent negative thoughts, feelings of guilt or shame, and a profound sense of disconnection from the world around them. Resulting signs and symptoms are not only emotional, they can also be physical

In their attempts to avoid social situations or events that might trigger their symptoms, our clients presenting with PTSD are often struggling with social isolation, which, in turn, may increase their vulnerability to depression. Even the smallest noise can trigger a heightened state of alertness, leading to hypervigilance, emotional turmoil, irritability, and difficulty concentrating. This is a natural response to being in a constant state of stress, where the body's exposure to stress-related chemicals reduces cognitive function. Further to this, our clients often present with sleep disturbances and distressing physical reactions like a racing heart, which reveals the chaos within. A protective dissociation may sometimes manifest as a feeling of detachment, leaving individuals feeling isolated, adrift in their own existence, wrestling with gaps in their memory.

Recognising what symptoms your client is experiencing, be they emotional, physical or behavioural, is paramount in the effective treatment of PTSD. In the initial session it is essential to help our clients articulate a specific goal for therapy. I often help them achieve this by thoroughly exploring the problematic symptoms they present with. This is often easier for our clients who may have little idea of what life will be like without the life impacting symptoms, particularly if they have been suffering with PTSD for a prolonged time. They may have a sense of hopelessness, and it is our job to begin the process of building an expectancy for change and better outcomes.

By addressing each symptom individually, I guide my clients to envision a world free from each individual symptom, and one by one we work through the list until we have a clear idea of what life will look like without these distressing experiences '*when the issue no longer exists*'. In this statement there is a presupposition that the issue *will* come to an end. In counselling, we refer to this technique as the "miracle question," while in hypnotherapy, it bears similarities to a "future pace."

The experiential task of fully embodying this future self as if it has already been achieved, is employed during trance and revisited repeatedly outside of sessions to counter any negative thoughts, feelings, or behaviours that may arise. When they do arise, and initially they probably will, they are noticed without judgement, challenged and replaced with a more solution directed self-narrative. The envisioned outcome when fully embodied by the client, allows them to connect emotionally and mentally with their desired future-self.

Within the therapeutic context, the power of hypnotherapy emerges as a remarkable tool; it can induce a profound state of relaxation, enabling individuals to feel grounded and at ease. A longer progressive muscle relaxation works well here with a deepener, and with some well-chosen and well-timed suggestions about the inevitability of change, may be as far as we get in a first session.

For many who have been existing in a hypervigilant state, relaxing can feel very unsafe and may not come easily, so even a light relaxation can be profound for them. Let's remember that these clients are wired for hypervigilance neurologically and physiologically. This may well be the first time in a very long time that they have been able to relax at all, so even moderate relaxation is a step in the right direction. I once had a client who could not close his eyes for more than a minute as this was not safe for him, he needed to keep his eyes on the door to be aware of any danger that may burst into the room. Therefore, we work within the limitations of how our clients present and make everything okay, no matter what. Be creative, be flexible, it is important to remember that any level of comfort or relaxation that these clients achieve is a success. Those who can achieve any degree of comfort are moving into a new state that not only mitigates their immediate distress, but it also forms a vital foundation for the intricate work that lies ahead. Through this safe, respectful journey our clients can begin to regain a feeling of agency and control, essential for fostering healing and transformation.

Once we have cultivated a strong rapport, established a safe environment, and imparted knowledge about the process of hypnotherapy to our clients, allowing them to experience relaxation, perhaps for the first time in a long time, we can turn our attention to the significance of incorporating homework techniques. These may include cognitive awareness exercises, challenging negative thought patterns, mindfulness practices, and self-hypnosis, all aimed at focusing on the client's specific solutions rather than dwelling on the problems themselves.

It is imperative when dealing with any client to never send them away from the consultation room without first equipping them with strategies to tackle their conscious state, this is perhaps even more important when dealing with a client with PTSD. Awareness is vital for managing the damaging subconscious routines and patterns our clients may be operating under, often without realising it. As hypnotherapists we all understand how powerful the subconscious mind is, and how it often runs patterns and habits without conscious awareness. However, when we bring these patterns into conscious awareness, we begin to cast a light on them that illuminates our ability to purposefully choose our next course of action. In effect we put our clients in the driver seat, it is then up to them to decide; what shall I do next?

I consistently remind every client, just as I would remind you now, that awareness is the cornerstone of transformation, and as we've explored in earlier chapters, repetition is the precursor of change. It can effectively stimulate neuroplasticity in the brain to establish new advantageous habits and patterns. As mentioned, few of the approaches I routinely implement with my clients involve cognitive and awareness-based methods. These complement the hypnotherapy sessions, empowering clients to identify and confront harmful thoughts, emotions, and beliefs that might have tethered them to their trauma. Subsequently, suggestions created from the changes that have been noted by our clients, and fed back to them in the trance state, acting as powerful persuaders that change is indeed occurring.

Cognitive-Behavioural hypnotherapy is a further step in merging these two modalities. By integrating cognitive-behavioural techniques with hypnotherapy, we focus on transforming negative thought patterns linked to the trauma. Each session commences with a dialogue about what the client has observed to have changed, what others have noticed and what they feel has shifted. Often we need to assist our clients to recognise the changes that are occurring as they may still be overly focused on that which is not working, instead of what is working. The changes therefore can often be hiding in plain sight and sometimes we just need to shine the light onto them. This newfound insight is fortified during hypnosis with suggestions such as, "As you become aware of more changes occurring each day, you might find yourself filled with anticipation for a future that aligns with your desires," or "The more you take control of your powerful thoughts, the more you are noticing… you are gaining control of all those other aspects of your life… ."

Mindfulness is also an important process to introduce to both the hypnotherapy session and to the between session conscious state. Clients are guided to be in present moment awareness, rather than being back in the past revisiting the trauma. Through awareness techniques they are taught how to bring themselves back from the catastrophic past or the imagined future, neither of which exists in the present moment, to be 'here and now'. During the hypnotherapy session our client's ability to notice, challenge and release unhelpful thoughts feelings and emotions are reinforced in the hypnotic state. Times that have been discussed, where they have been able to do just that, are introduced as hypnotic convincers and enhance their ability to continue to step out of stress into the calm.

Breath work is also an essential part of this process again reinforced in trance, our clients are taught how to connect to the exhalation, by making it longer and deeper than usual and to release any muscular tightness, particularly from the shoulders, neck or anywhere they hold on to tension as they exhale. These two physiological actions send a message to the body of safety. Parasympathetic nervous system is then activated as the client steps out of stress mode into calm. Practiced in the hypnotic induction, our clients have the ability, under our guidance, to fully embody this experience. All of these techniques have the ability to enhance our client's emotional regulation and move them toward beneficial change.

It is essential to guide clients to notice even the smallest changes in their symptoms. Perhaps introducing journaling can serve as a tangible form of evidence, allowing them to track their progress on the path to healing. By noting how often they are triggered, the duration of these episodes, and the intensity of their feelings, clients can begin to see that positive change is indeed occurring. This realisation acts as a powerful motivator, encouraging them to persevere with their therapeutic work. When presented at the next session, this information and the changes noted are introduced as therapeutic suggestions readily accepted by the client's subconscious mind.

With this foundation firmly laid, we then turn our focus to reprocessing traumatic memories. Within the depths of the subconscious, memories of trauma can become "stuck," replaying with the same intensity as when the events first unfolded. When a client expresses that it feels as though the trauma occurred yesterday, it indicates that the memory has been stored in a region of the brain associated with rapid retrieval. This phenomenon is linked to the amygdala, a crucial area for processing emotions and storing traumatic memories, which serves to keep individuals hyper-vigilant in the face of potential danger (van der Kolk, 2014). This response is the body's way of ensuring readiness to confront the same threat should it arise again.

Hypnotherapy offers a pathway to reprocess these memories, enabling clients to approach their experiences with a greater sense of emotional detachment. Techniques such as Visual Kinaesthetic Dissociation, age regression, guided visualisation, and reframing can help clients re-contextualise their trauma, thereby diminishing its emotional impact.

Through the skilful application of hypnotherapy, we also aim to desensitise the damaging cycle of recurring triggers that often arise from trauma. Triggers, be they sights, sounds, smells, or particular situations often weave a complex web within the subconscious, eliciting automatic fight-or-flight responses. Hypnotherapy can be used effectively to diminish the intensity of these triggers, allowing clients to approach previously anxiety-inducing stimuli or situations with a sense of calm, rather than fear.

Another crucial step in the therapeutic process is the empowerment of the client. Individuals grappling with PTSD frequently experience a profound sense of powerlessness. Hypnotherapy highlights and nurtures the client's inherent capacity for self-directed healing and thereby empowers the client to be an active participant in their own recovery journey. This reinforces their sense of mastery over both mind and body.

During the therapeutic intervention phase of hypnosis, clients are guided to safely reprocess the trauma by firstly establishing a safe space and through the use of imagery, identifying and connecting to coping strategies, or empowering scenarios, such as past accomplishments of overcoming challenges. The use of metaphor and story can aid in processing and reframing past traumatic events. Negative beliefs linked to the trauma are identified, challenged and reframed into something more acceptable to the client through a process of incorporating the knowledge and wisdom of the present-self, that the past-self did not yet possess. Emotional regulation strategies are taught to manage anxiety and stress in the waking states and positive outcomes of these strategies are sought out, affirmed and reinforced in subsequent hypnotherapy sessions.

Future-pacing and visualisation exercises are incorporated to assist the client to focus their attention on their intention to be healed by envisaging an empowered future, acknowledging changes that have occurred as convincers on which to build an expectancy of even more change, subsequently reinforcing all positive behaviours. At the conclusion of the session, clients are provided with post-hypnotic suggestions aimed at acknowledging and reinforcing therapeutic benefits and enhancing their coping strategies in response to triggers, followed by a gradual return to full alertness.

Regular follow-up sessions are scheduled to monitor progress and adjust techniques, enhancing the healing process. As rapport continues to build, supported by therapeutic successes, clients continue to experience hypnosis in a safe way. Other strategies may be introduced designed to de-traumatise the initiating event. Importantly this can be done in a content free way if it is too traumatic for the client to revisit the trauma.

Dissociative techniques are also powerful tools used in hypnosis for addressing PTSD. These methods facilitate the processing of traumatic memories while minimising emotional distress during therapy, Visual–Kinaesthetic Dissociation (VKD) is one such technique.

VKD is specifically designed to help individuals reprocess traumatic memories without experiencing overwhelming emotions, and is a therapeutic tool designed to help people step back from traumatic or emotionally charged memories. Instead of re-experiencing the memory with full emotional intensity, VKD guides the person to "watch" the memory as though it were a film, separating the visual experience of seeing the event, from the kinaesthetic experience of feeling the emotions in the body.

A Rewind Technique is one example of VKD. These techniques offer structured approaches to managing traumatic memories by encouraging dissociation from the trauma itself. Initially, it aids clients in separating from the emotional and physical sensations linked to the traumatic memory, facilitated by inducing a hypnotic state of relaxation. This allows clients to observe the memory in a calm state and from a safe distance, avoiding the need to relive it. Through safe visualisation, clients are guided to view the memory in a disassociated way, such as if projected on a screen or even through a process of double dissociation, where they envisage watching themselves viewing the memory whilst deeply relaxed. This creates a mental detachment, enabling them to replay the traumatic event in a secure and controlled way while keeping an emotional distance.

During the process, clients are encouraged to alter the visual aspects of the memory. By manipulating elements such as speed, fast-forwarding or rewinding until it becomes a mere fleeting flash, as they transition from one secure point before the event to another safe point afterwards. Adjustments in colours, sounds, or feelings associated with the memory further help reduce its emotional grip, reframing the memory as they experience reviewing it whilst being completely calm. This helps the brain to recognise the memory as now nonthreatening, and associated fear or anxiety are diminished.

The technique concludes with integration, future pacing and closure. After reprocessing the memory, clients visualise themselves in a future free from the old response patterns, reinforcing positive emotions and further facilitating the integration of the altered experience which significantly contributes to emotional healing.

Research increasingly supports the efficacy of the Rewind Technique as a treatment for PTSD, demonstrating robust evidence through rigorous scientific methods. Notably, a recent randomised controlled trial (RCT) conducted remotely via video calls found that the Rewind Technique produced a large effect size in reducing PTSD symptoms, comparable in impact to more established therapies such as trauma-focused cognitive behavioural therapy (CBT-TF) and eye movement desensitisation and reprocessing (EMDR), but with fewer sessions and potentially greater cost-efficiency (Astill Wright L. et al., 2023).

The study involved 40 participants and showed maintained symptom improvement up to 16 weeks post-treatment, indicating sustained benefits. The mechanism behind the Rewind Technique, involving dissociation from traumatic memories, safe visualisation, alteration of memory imagery, and integration in a calming environment, appears to underpin its effectiveness by enabling clients to reprocess trauma safely and reduce its emotional intensity.

Practitioners have long observed the fast and painless nature of VKD techniques such as the Rewind Technique, with anecdotal reports of fast relief from panic, flashbacks, and anxiety after as little as just one session, adding experiential weight alongside clinical trials (Human Givens Institute, 2024). Collectively, these findings offer strong empirical backing to the technique's use in trauma therapy and suggest it may become an increasingly recognised option within clinical psychology and hypnotherapy practices.

Both the Rewind Technique and dissociative techniques play essential roles in hypnosis for PTSD. By allowing clients to dissociate from traumatic memories and process them in a safe, controlled manner, these approaches promote healing and emotional regulation. Incorporating these techniques into therapy can empower clients to reclaim their narratives and enhance their overall well-being. If you are not using the Visual Kinaesthetic Dissociation techniques, I thoroughly recommend you seek out a reputable course.

Research also underscores the effectiveness of hypnotherapy in general as a complementary treatment for PTSD. Cardeña and Spiegel's (1991) illustrated that hypnosis can substantially alleviate PTSD symptoms, especially when used alongside other therapeutic methods. Hypnotherapy's capacity to reduce arousal, improve emotional regulation, and facilitate cognitive restructuring renders it particularly suitable for trauma treatment.

Furthermore, hypnosis has been observed to significantly diminish flashbacks, nightmares, and hyperarousal symptoms in PTSD patients due to the ability to access the subconscious mind allowing for a more profound and expedited processing of traumatic memories compared to traditional talk therapy.

Case Study: Mark's Journey Toward Healing

Mark, a 36-year-old ambulance paramedic, sought hypnotherapy after experiencing severe PTSD following his team being called to a building collapse three years earlier. Despite valiant attempts to save all the casualties, paramedics were unable to do so. A small child Mark was trying to save tragically died from his injuries before he could be freed from the rubble. Mark was haunted by vivid flashbacks, unable to sleep and felt that his life was spiralling out of control. Traditional therapy had helped to some degree, but he remained stuck in a cycle of fear and avoidance that spilled out into all areas of his life.

After all the preliminary pre talk and education had been conducted, Mark was guided into a state of deep relaxation. During his first experience of hypnotherapy a safe space was established and suggestions for change and the powerful connection between his mind and body were given. It is important to match the timing of these suggestions with the gentle micro-movements of his body as he gently releases observable muscular tightness and tension. Relaxing suggestions are also timed with the exhalation, the body's natural relaxation response. Observation of our clients is of prime importance during these sessions.

During the second hypnotic session, and only after good rapport had been established, guided Visual Kinaesthetic Dissociation techniques were utilised. Mark was able to revisit the memory of the collapse, importantly, not to relive it, rather to observe it from a very safe and detached perspective. Over several sessions utilising VKD techniques, as mentioned previously in this chapter, Mark was able to reframe the event, shifting his perspective from feelings of helplessness to recognising his bravery and his efforts to save lives. The "safe space" of his mind, created in hypnotherapy became a sanctuary he could return to whenever he felt overwhelmed. Combined with the cognitive techniques discussed in this chapter, Mark was able to observe his triggers had lost their power to control him, and he began to reclaim his life. Within three months, Mark reported significant improvements in his sleep, mood, and ability to return to work.

In summary, hypnotherapy is a transformative tool for individuals suffering from PTSD. By accessing the subconscious mind, it enables clients to process trauma, break free from triggers, and reclaim control over their lives. Through compassionate guidance, hypnotherapists empower clients to turn their pain into a source of strength and healing.

As research continues to validate its effectiveness, hypnotherapy provides hope for those seeking relief from the lasting impacts of trauma. For clients like Mark, and countless others, hypnotherapy offers not just recovery but the possibility of reclaiming the life they once lived.

It is important, as it is for all our clients, to tailor each session to the individual's needs. It is never a one size fits all solution and by recognising that every client's experience of trauma is unique, we place ourselves in the best position to help. Techniques such as ego strengthening, future pacing, dissociative techniques, post-hypnotic suggestions, mindfulness and cognitive reframing tools are integral in this approach, ensuring clients leave sessions with practical tools essential for ongoing resilience.

Chapter Twenty-Six

TRANSFORMING PHOBIAS THROUGH HYPNOTHERAPY

Phobias are a very common presentation seen in hypnotherapy practice. Any therapist who has been practicing for some time will have encountered a wide range of phobias, some more familiar, such as fear of heights (acrophobia) or spiders (arachnophobia) or flying (aviophobia), and others are more unusual, such as an intense fear of birds, butterflies, clowns or even balloons. By their nature, phobias are rooted in the subconscious mind, which means they often defy logical explanation. The person is usually well aware that their fear is disproportionate, yet the overwhelming anxiety persists regardless of rational thought. According to Health Direct Australia, a phobia is defined as an extreme fear of something that is out of proportion to the threat posed and causes distress that greatly affects your life and leads to you actively avoiding the object or situation.

Consider, for example, a client who presents with an intense fear of butterflies. Consciously, they know that butterflies are harmless creatures, admired by many for their beauty. Yet each encounter triggers an overwhelming fear response, racing heart, shallow breathing, and a need to escape. Through regression work, such a fear might trace back to an early childhood experience: perhaps being startled when a butterfly suddenly flew close to their face during a moment when they already felt unsafe. Research continues to show that many phobias can be linked to early traumatic or distressing experiences where, as children, individuals did not yet possess the emotional resources to manage or process the event adequately. At such a young age, they lacked the emotional resources to make sense of the experience. The subconscious mind therefore stores the image and memory as threatening. Decades later, the body still reacts as if the fluttering butterfly presents a danger, even though the conscious mind knows otherwise.

Because phobias originate in the subconscious part of the mind, hypnotherapy can be a particularly effective tool. As we know, the hypnotic state allows clients to bypass the conscious, rational mind and access the deeper roots of the phobia. Regression work is especially useful here, as it can enable a safe exploration of the original sensitising event that may have triggered the fear.

Safety is once again the critical aspect of this therapy. As with all regression work, it is vital that client safety is paramount. Revisiting the origin of a phobia can sometimes bring the client close to past trauma. In these situations, dissociative techniques can be utilised during regression to provide a safe framework: the client can then observe the event from a safe distance, rather than re-experiencing it. This approach allows for integration without re-traumatisation.

Regression can also be combined with inner child work in such situations, giving clients access to resources and coping strategies they did not possess at the time of the original event. From this perspective, the past can be reframed through the lens of present strengths, creating an opportunity for healing. Hypnotherapy uniquely incorporates reframing techniques, often paired with metaphors, ego strengthening, and positive hypnotic suggestions, to enhance a client's ability to tackle challenges and overcome obstacles. These metaphors aid in reprocessing memories, modifying their storage and reducing the intensity of phobic responses. The client is then guided through future pacing to a future where the Phobic response no longer exists, allowing them to embody a more resourceful version of themselves and envision experiencing life without the phobia. This therapeutic process links closely to the principles of cognitive restructuring. Hypnosis enhances the capacity for cognitive restructuring by creating a state where initial traumatic imprints can be safely challenged and reframed (Alladin, 2016).

Neuroscientific studies support this process, showing that traumatic memories are typically encoded and reinforced in the amygdala and hippocampus, regions of the brain associated with fear conditioning and memory consolidation. When memories are revisited and reprocessed in a safe therapeutic context, they can reconsolidate differently, often becoming less emotionally charged and more adaptive.

Taken together, these findings give weight to the premiss that hypnotherapy, particularly when utilising regression, dissociation, inner child work, and reframing techniques, provides an effective pathway for helping clients with phobias. By addressing the subconscious roots of the phobia and allowing for the memory to be reprocessed and stored in less distressing ways, hypnotherapy supports both symptom relief and deep emotional healing.

Research supports hypnotherapy's use as a powerful and evolving tool for addressing fear and phobias, providing strong empirical support for its efficacy. Fuhr et al. (2023) conducted a rater-blind, randomised controlled pilot trial evaluating individual outpatient hypnotherapy (8–12 sessions) versus a waitlist control in patients with agoraphobia and found that hypnotherapy produced significantly greater reductions in agoraphobic/anxiety symptoms, with low dropout, high patient satisfaction, and no serious adverse events, supporting its feasibility, safety, and preliminary efficacy.

Another study found that just two hypnotherapy sessions over four meetings led to a significant 51.87% reduction in phobia symptoms, evidencing its rapid and effective impact (Wijaya & Trini, 2023). Additionally, modern approaches integrating hypnotherapy with innovative technologies such as Virtual Reality (VR) are being studied with promising results. They are seen to enhance exposure therapy in a safe, controlled environment showing improving outcomes in phobia treatment. For our clients who find it difficult to visualise this could be helpful, however I would postulate that as hypnotherapists we already allow our clients to enter a virtual reality of their own making.

In 2024, Rosendahl, Alldredge, and Haddenhorst conducted a comprehensive systematic review of 49 meta-analyses covering 261 randomised controlled trials and found consistent evidence that hypnosis is effective for a range of mental and somatic health issues. Effects were at least medium for over half of outcomes, with particular strength for pain management, medical procedures and paediatric applications, and significant benefits for anxiety and depressive symptoms. The review also indicates hypnosis can be comparable to established treatments such as cognitive behavioural therapy, with some studies reporting faster anxiety relief mid-treatment.

Overall, current evidence supports hypnotherapy as an effective, adaptable modality for treating anxiety, fear and phobias, with ongoing research expanding its applications and refining its integration with other therapeutic techniques.

CASE STUDY: LAYLA

Layla, a 15-year-old girl, came to hypnotherapy because of an intense avian phobia which was significantly affecting her life. The mere sight of a bird would trigger waves of panic, making it impossible for her to walk outside when birds were nesting in Spring or even stay in a room with a caged bird. Initially, Layla managed this phobia by avoiding situations where birds might be present. However, she revealed that her phobia was progressively worsening, which is not uncommon. When we consider the principles of neuroplasticity and habit formation, we recall that the human brain is adept at creating and maintaining habits, regardless of whether they are beneficial or detrimental. Consequently, Layla's phobia was intensifying, and an upcoming school trip to the

Healesville Sanctuary, to study birds of prey was causing her severe anxiety.

In our first session, Layla shared her apprehensions about the upcoming excursion, revealing that her fear extended beyond birds to include the possibility of losing control and panicking in front of her peers. The thought of such a public display and the potential reactions from her classmates heightened her anxiety. With this insight, we embarked on a journey to free her from this paralysing fear.

Using gentle regression, I guided Layla to the root of her fear by reconnecting her with the emotion linked to the issue at hand. It's important to note that I did not explicitly mention her bird phobia. This choice of language is crucial because the subconscious mind doesn't operate logically or literally, meaning the original triggering event might not relate to birds at all. In Layla's case, it was related, but I've had clients with issues like a physical verbal tic that, when traced back, stemmed from a fear of their mother's death. This serves as a reminder: we must not lead clients in a direction we believe is right, as it might inadvertently steer them away from the real issue. Instead, we allow them to guide the process, using open-ended, non-leading questions to help them discover their own solutions.

As the scene unfolded through her words, we returned to the autumn morning when, at the tender age of three, she was chased by a goose at a children's farm. Her tiny legs struggled to outrun the honking monster, and her heart pounded louder in her chest than the flapping wings behind her. This memory, buried for years, resurfaced with clarity just as though it happened yesterday.

In the realm of hypnotherapy, Layla was able to transform the experience using present-day wisdom, knowing that she was safe, and the bird could not harm her. We played the image back and forward faster and faster, giving the goose a handbag and an old-fashioned bonnet, and a silly jacket, just like mother goose who was only protecting her babies. The image became funny as mother goose flapped around faster and faster while the goslings looked on confused and Layla began to laugh. Within the safe confines of her subconscious mind, we replayed the memory with a new narrative. The goose, once a giant foe, became merely a curious creature, driven by its instinct to protect her young.

"Now, imagine feeling empowered. Really connect to the feeling of confidence just as you've felt many times before." I suggested, "Walk past the birds at the farm feeling that confidence now you have a new understanding of what that was all about, just a mother protecting her young"

Next, we employed desensitisation techniques to help Layla review this experience without emotional triggering. Gradually, through guided imagery, she visualised scenarios with birds at a safe distance, turning her fear into familiarity. Over successive sessions, we edged closer until she could, in her mind, sit calmly in their presence.

Future pacing became a pivotal part of our work. Layla visualised herself participating in the school excursion, walking gracefully through any aviary feeling empowered and confident, engaging with school activities easily and effortlessly. Importantly she visualised herself arriving home after the excursion, telling her mother how well she had gone, and how comfortable she had felt. She was then invited to embody the feelings of relief and pride for how she had experienced the day in such an empowered way. This forward-looking perspective enabled Layla to emotionally connect to her new experience in the present moment, as her physiology and neurology simultaneously adjusted to her optimal outcome as if she had already experienced it, effectively rewiring her for success.

Finally, post-hypnotherapeutic suggestions bridged the gap between her subconscious realisations and daily life. We fortified her new perspective with affirmations of strength and calm, echoing the beneficial changes in her mind. Layla emerged not only anticipating freedom from her phobia but embodying it as she actually began to look forward to the excursion.

In conclusion, Layla's eventual journey to the Sanctuary became more than an excursion; it was a testament to her inner strength and resilience. Hypnotherapy did not merely soothe her fears, rather it empowered Layla to safely confront and reinterpret them. This allowed Layla to create a future where she was no longer tethered to the ghosts of past traumas and liberate herself so she could experience more empowered outcomes.

Chapter Twenty-Seven

UNLOCKING PEAK POTENTIAL – HYPNOTHERAPY FOR PERFORMANCE ENHANCEMENT

Does success have a mental edge, and if so, how do we access it to achieve our best performances? What separates the good from the great in any field? Of course, we all know that physical ability, talent, and preparation are vital in achieving success, however we see time and time again that what often separates the good from the great is the unseen, the mental edge. Hypnotherapy serves as a powerful tool for performance enhancement across various domains, including sports, business, academics, and creative pursuits. By accessing the subconscious mind, hypnotherapy helps individuals overcome self-doubt, by quietening the negative inner voice that tells you," I can't", I'll never" or "I'm just not good enough." This makes space for our clients to access the immense power of their mind to focus their attention on their intention to be something more or to achieve something more.

As performance coach Tony Robbins states, "The only thing that's keeping you from getting what you want is the story you keep telling yourself."

This chapter explores how hypnotherapy can optimise performance, the mechanisms behind its effectiveness, and practical applications to help you unlock your full potential.

Throughout this book we have talked a great deal about harnessing the power of the mind and body to work together to achieve different outcomes. This is no different, when we seek to achieve peak performances, we must begin with the mind. Research indicates that mental conditioning and visualisation techniques can significantly improve outcomes. As we hypnotherapists know, the brain often cannot distinguish between vividly imagined experiences and actual events. Therefore, as discussed in previous chapters, rehearsing success mentally can condition both the mind and body for optimal performance.

Hypnotherapy amplifies this principle, by creating the neurological changes that have been discussed in Chapter 6. The Brain in Trance. When working with the subconscious mind, which governs habits, automatic responses, and deeply ingrained beliefs, it's crucial to envision the desired outcomes. This may sound simple, but is often challenging, as our clients will be used to seeking out and focusing on all the parts of their performance that they dislike the most. The corrected imaginative process, of focusing on what they wish to achieve, helps align the subconscious with success, often leading to transformative results. Interestingly, the manner in which clients engage in this imaginative activity is flexible and varies individually.

Visual individuals might utilise images, colours, and shapes, while other clients might rely on auditory senses, engaging with sounds, words, and rhythms. Additionally, some may connect through movement and touch, or through olfactory, gustatory, vestibular, or interoceptive experiences, involving smell, taste, balance, spatial orientation, or internal bodily sensations such as hunger, heartbeat, and breathing. How ever your client connects to their imaginative potential is fine, the important thing is that they can get a sense of their success in a way that works for them.

In the realm of performance enhancement, hypnotherapy plays a pivotal role by working intricately with the subconscious mind, which governs habits, automatic responses, and deeply ingrained beliefs. Therefore, understanding the importance of focusing on the desired outcomes is paramount, as this imaginative technique helps synchronise the subconscious with success, often resulting in transformative changes.

As with all other issues we have dealt with, it is essential to prepare our clients for success, by exploring the past to ensure there are no anchors that are preventing them from moving forward. Therefore, past traumas, or limiting beliefs need to be explored and reframed to ensure the path is clear to freely move forward without restriction. This clearance is akin to removing weeds from a garden bed before planting the new crop.

Cognitive awareness techniques are also taught and employed by our clients to allow for them to notice and intercept any old repetitive thought, habit or pattern that will otherwise lead straight back to the old problem. Once the past is cleared, we are free to look to the future through the lens of the present moment. By this I mean that we can get our clients to fully associate with their future state as if they have already achieved it, a powerful future pace!

Hypnotherapy's application in performance enhancement is notably diverse. Our aim is to assist our clients in overcoming mental barriers such as performance anxiety, fear of failure or negative self-talk. We reframe these limitations and redirect their focus toward a more positive narrative and a more empowering mindset. Old beliefs such as "I'm not good enough" or "I'll fail" are replaced with more positive success orientated affirmations such as "I am capable" or "I can succeed." This combined with a daily self-hypnotic practice, where our clients completely associate with their success state, by stepping right into it as though they have already achieved it, for a few minutes each day will assist in rewiring the brain to support the successful outcome.

Hypnotherapy also has the ability to facilitate a state of flow which enhances our client's ability to focus and concentrate, which in turn allows distractions to diminish, enabling our clients to fully engage with their tasks. We ask our clients to mentally rehearse their successful performances over and over again. Athletes may imagine crossing the finish line first or achieving a personal best outcome, performers may imagine a standing ovation, and professionals may picture delivering outstanding presentations.

I have seen many golfers who imagined their best golf swing, and surfers who imagined catching the perfect wave. No matter what our clients are wanting to achieve, we need to listen to their language and the phrases they use that are meaningful to them. Therefore, it is not necessary for us to know what a perfect golf swing, or the perfect wave looks like or feels like, because our clients already do.

Hypnosis also has the ability to bolster confidence by embedding affirmations like "my body knows what to do," "I've done it before, and I can do it again" or "I perform at my best when I stop thinking about it and get into the flow." I have had many clients saying, I kept hearing your voice in my head stating a positive suggestion such as "You can do it, when you believe you can, you will" which significantly bolsters self-confidence. Moreover, hypnosis reduces stress and anxiety by calming the nervous system and reducing cortisol levels, promoting relaxation and enabling performance free from the hindrance of stress.

Numerous studies support the efficacy of hypnosis for performance enhancement. Zhao and Liu (2022) reviewed the use of hypnosis in sport and concluded that, when used in addition to conventional training, hypnosis reliably enhanced psychological factors, reducing competitive anxiety, improving concentration, and bolstering self-confidence. Not surprisingly, these factors underpin performance gains. It was also reported that these cognitive improvements translated into measurable benefits in skill acquisition and task execution. Hypnosis that was individually tailored to the athlete yielded the most benefits when delivered over repeated sessions. Here again we see the importance of repetition.

In the real world we now see that many athletes, including Olympic gold medallists, are utilising hypnosis to refine their performance and importantly strengthen their mindset, in order to optimise their results. Furthermore, research demonstrates that hypnosis can effectively enhance performance not only by boosting confidence, reducing stress as mentioned above, but also it can improve problem-solving abilities in both professional and academic settings.

Hypnotherapy is a gateway to peak performance. By removing mental blocks, reinforcing positive beliefs, and aligning the subconscious with success, it empowers individuals to achieve their best, enabling our clients to rewrite their story and step into the excellence they are capable of achieving. However, as with any therapeutic approach, hypnotherapy for performance enhancement needs to be client-centred and ethically focused. We must take care to avoid creating unrealistic expectations or reinforcing perfectionism, which in itself is a problem. Instead, we aim to build resilience, self-belief, and sustainable strategies for success.

CASE STUDY: MIA, THE CONCERT PIANIST

Mia, a 27-year-old professional pianist, sought hypnotherapy after experiencing debilitating stage fright before performances. Despite years of training, she frequently doubted her abilities and often felt her hands tremble on stage.

During her initial hypnotherapy session, we delved into the root of Mia's fear. Through hypnosis, she recalled a childhood recital where she went blank and could not complete part of her piece. She felt humiliated, as her family and those who she greatly respected were all watching on. Each time she took to the stage since that time, the same familiar feeling of foreboding overcame her. The subconscious memory, which had been stored in that part of her brain that enables easy access as a protective mechanism had carried over into her adult life and quickly resurfaced before every performance. According to Mia, it was getting worse. This is a common occurrence. The human mind loves a habit and as we know the subconscious mind is wonderfully good at running habits and does not discern between a helpful habit or an unhelpful one. Therefore, again we see the principle of 'what we repeat and what we focus on we strengthen,' in Mia's predictable outcomes.

During regression Mia was able to reshape this memory, enabling her to realise that a single childhood mistake did not define her or determine her talent or future performances. She was able to address her faulty beliefs with a combination of cognitive behavioural hypnotherapy transforming her belief that she would certainly "mess up again" to "I've practised hard, and I trust myself to perform well."

In subsequent sessions, and through self-hypnotic daily practice, Mia rehearsed her performances in a hypnotic state, envisioning herself playing with ease, confidence, and joy, culminating in a standing ovation from the audience.

After several sessions Mia reported feeling significantly calmer, her confidence grew, and she began to enjoy her performances once again.

Chapter Twenty-Eight

HYPNOTHERAPY FOR FUNCTIONAL NEUROLOGICAL DISORDERS: UNLOCKING NEURO-PHYSIOLOGICAL HEALING.

Functional Neurological Disorders (FND) are frequently misunderstood, often misdiagnosed, and exist at the complex intersection between mind, brain and body. For individuals experiencing FND, symptoms such as seizures, paralysis, tremors, walking difficulties, confusion and memory issues, numbness or loss of sensation, speech, swallowing and concentration difficulties are common, disturbing and profoundly real.

Many other neurological conditions have identifiable structural causes, such as tumours or lesions, making them easier to identify. FND, on the other hand, emerges from disruptions in the sending and receiving of signals in the brain's communication pathways. These disruptions reflect the intricate interplay between psychological and neurological processes.

There is a recognised connection between FND and the associated presenting symptoms; Functional Neurological Symptoms (FNS) and trauma. Individuals experiencing FNS often have a history of psychological trauma or significant stressors. According to the American Psychological Association (APA), traumatic experiences can alter brain function and may precipitate or exacerbate the symptoms of FNS (American Psychological Association, 2023). This connection underscores the importance of considering psychological factors and past trauma when diagnosing and treating FNS, highlighting the need for therapies that address both the psychological and physiological aspects of the disorder.

Hypnotherapy is rapidly gaining recognition as a powerful therapeutic tool for tackling FND or FNS, thanks to its unique ability to engage the subconscious mind and transform entrenched neurological patterns. Unlike more mainstream therapies, such as physiotherapy and occupational therapy, which primarily address only the physical symptoms of FND, hypnotherapy delves deeper, getting to the root cause by addressing both the physiological and psychological underpinnings. This dual focus makes hypnotherapy an effective approach for paving the way towards relief, understanding, and healing.

For the purpose of this writing, I will refer to both FND and FNS under the single term "Functional Neurological Disorder" FND to encompass the condition and its associated symptoms collectively.

In this chapter, we will explore the nature of FND, delve into the neuroscience underpinning its symptoms, and examine how hypnotherapy facilitates healing. Through research insights and case studies, the profound potential of this approach will be illustrated.

~

As always, we need to have a good understanding of a condition if we wish to effectively assist our clients in achieving symptom relief. Therefore, let's look a little deeper at FND and how it presents significant challenges in diagnosis and treatment.

Many individuals with FND undergo extensive medical testing, often only to hear that their symptoms lack organic explanations, in layman's terms, they are told, "there is nothing wrong with you." Worse still, many are informed, "it's all in your mind." If you have ever found yourself in this situation, you will be very aware that being treated like this can lead to heartache, frustration, stigma, and a deep sense of invalidation. As a hypnotherapist however, I welcome clients who have been thoroughly medically evaluated, with any underlying pathology ruled out. When they tell me, "They say it's all in my mind." I'm hopeful. For me, this is a positive statement that can be utilised to reinforce to the client how amazingly powerful their mind is. When we harness that ability and channel it in a different direction, imagine what could be possible. When we know for sure all physical underlying causes have already been ruled out it is an optimal starting point. As hypnotherapists we recognise the mind's immense power and potential, therefore this is an area where hypnotherapy can truly make a difference.

In recent years, our understanding of the brain has significantly advanced, and neuroscience has clarified that FND is no longer simply considered to be a collection of "imaginary" symptoms. Rather, it is a disorder of function where the brain's ability to send and interpret signals is disrupted. With the advent of functional MRI (fMRI), we can now observe the functioning brain in real-time, measuring brain activity, blood flow, and examining areas involved in specific cognitive tasks, emotions, and sensory processes. This makes fMRI an invaluable tool for understanding FND. Observations during symptom expression have revealed altered activity in specific brain regions, including the prefrontal cortex, limbic system, and sensorimotor areas, now known to be implicated in FND.

As noted earlier, FND is frequently linked with psychological factors like trauma, stress, or anxiety. These elements can act as triggers for clients or as influencing factors that sustain or reinforce maladaptive neural patterns and strengthen a cycle of dysfunction.

Hypnotherapy is particularly suited to address FND due to its dual engagement with both the mind and body. By inducing a trance state, a condition of focused attention and heightened suggestibility, hypnotherapy allows therapists to access the subconscious, enabling engagement with the neural circuits involved in FND and promote new patterns of functioning.

Let's review what happens in the brain of someone with FND. The Default Mode Network (DMN) in the brain, which is linked to self-focused type thinking, often becomes overly active in people with FND. This overactivity can lead individuals to dwell on or fixate excessively on their symptoms. Hypnosis plays a valuable role by reducing the DMN's activity, helping clients to move away from these unhealthy thought patterns.

FND symptoms can also worsen due to chronic stress affecting the Hypothalamic-Pituitary-Adrenal (HPA) axis. As we have previously observed, hypnosis aids in stress regulation by promoting relaxation and lowering cortisol levels, which in turn soothes the HPA axis and reduces the body's stress-related effects. Additionally, FND involves disruptions in communication between the brain's motor and sensory areas. Hypnosis assists in rebuilding these connections by using guided imagery and suggestions to stimulate both sensory and motor functions, aiding in more integrated brain performance.

Therefore, when we combine our knowledge of the neurology of FND and the neurology of trance discussed in chapter 6, The Brain in Trance: The Neuroscience of Hypnotherapy, we may begin to understand how hypnotherapy can harness the brain's natural ability to reorganise itself by forming new neural connections. For individuals with FND, this means establishing alternative pathways to override dysfunctional signalling and restore normal function.

The subconscious mind also plays a vital role in how FND symptoms manifest. For many individuals, these symptoms can emerge as reactions to unresolved trauma or emotional conflicts that have been suppressed by the conscious mind. Hypnotherapy offers a safe environment to delve into these subconscious processes, allowing for the exploration and redefinition of the emotional narratives that underpin the symptoms.

Imagine a client facing functional paralysis; they might uncover that their symptoms began following a time of intense stress or profound loss. Hypnotherapy serves as a bridge to this awareness, enabling them to process deep-seated emotions, reshape their relationship with the past, and gradually reduce the brain's tendency to produce symptoms that, although typically protective, may still be trying to address problems that have long since vanished. It's essential to remember that the subconscious mind lacks logical reasoning and literal interpretation. As a result, the symptoms or compulsions it presents might seem inexplicable when placed under conscious scrutiny, with resolutions and healing to be found only deep within the subconscious's hidden realms.

Now let's look at how we address FND clients, bearing in mind there is never a one size fits all panacea method. Successfully working with FND, as with all our clients, requires a multifaceted and individualised therapeutic approach. Below I have outlined some key hypnotherapy techniques used to tackle this disorder.

As stress or overwhelm often serve as significant triggers for FND symptoms, once again we see that prioritising relaxation and stress reduction is essential. This emphasis needs to extend beyond the therapy sessions, highlighting the importance of providing clients with effective tools to manage stress at home, reinforcing these skills between sessions. As reiterated throughout this book, combining these practices with cognitive tools enables clients to recognise unhelpful thoughts and emotions, allowing them to shift their focus towards desired outcomes, thus enhancing and promoting the neural plasticity of change.

Our hypnotherapy sessions usually begin by guiding clients into a state of deep relaxation, transitioning their nervous system from a fight-or-flight mode to a rest-and-digest state. This not only alleviates immediate symptoms but also lays the foundation for more profound therapeutic work. These practices continue through homework tasks that clients undertake daily, further enhancing neuroplasticity and fostering a solution-focused mindset.

Guided imagery is a crucial component both in sessions and at home. This technique engages the brain's sensory and motor pathways, assisting in retraining the brain to restore normal functioning. For example, a client with functional tremors might visualise their hands as steady and calm, reinforcing this imagery through repeated sessions. It's vital for clients to understand that they are active participants in this process, as the principle of repeated practice and immersion in the desired state strengthens the response of the brain and subconscious mind.

As mentioned, many clients with FND have experienced unresolved trauma. Hypnosis enables them to revisit these memories in a controlled, safe and supportive environment, processing the emotions tied to these experiences and reframing their impact. Once we have laid the foundational groundwork mentioned above and prepared our clients for ongoing success, we can then safely explore the past through methods like Age Regression, Visual Kinaesthetic Dissociation (VKD) and trauma reprocessing.

You may recall VKD as mentioned in previous chapters is an umbrella term for a group of techniques specifically designed to help individuals reprocess traumatic memories without experiencing overwhelming emotions. It is a therapeutic process designed to help people step back from traumatic or emotionally charged memories. Instead of re-experiencing the memory with full emotional intensity, VKD guides the person to "watch" the memory as though it were a film, separating the visual experience of seeing the event, from the kinaesthetic experience of feeling the emotions in the body.

There are many such techniques designed to facilitate visual-kinaesthetic dissociation, each offering unique ways to reduce the emotional impact of distressing memories or traumas. The Rewind Technique is one such technique frequently used. It involves mentally reversing and fast forwarding through a troubling event, often visualised as a film played backwards and forwards in a safe, controlled setting. Double Dissociation enhances this by encouraging individuals to watch themselves from a distance, as the observer, further reducing emotional intensity. The Fast Phobia Cure rapidly processes phobias by having the client envision the event in black and white, often at an accelerated speed. The Cinema Screen Technique, allows clients to project memories onto an imagined screen, allowing alteration of colours and sounds to lessen emotional reactions. The Observer Technique enables individuals to step outside themselves and view experiences from a detached, third-person perspective. Timeline techniques involve visualising life's events along a timeline, enabling clients to "float" above and view them with detachment.

I encourage you to learn whatever VKD technique that calls to you, if you have not already done so. They can be incredibly powerful in assisting our clients to feel empowered as they reframe their experiences from a safe distance and reclaim a sense of emotional resilience and healing.

In our work with clients, we seamlessly blend skilfully crafted direct and indirect suggestions with various techniques to foster healing and well-being. During hypnosis, suggestions are tailored to address the client's specific symptoms. Direct suggestions for someone with a hand tremor might include statements such as "each day you notice more and more how you can relax your hand and enjoy that stillness," while indirect suggestions may utilise metaphor and storytelling to inspire subconscious change.

A crucial component of the therapeutic process is future-pacing, which involves guiding the client to envision a future where they can embody an empowered state of health and confidence. This technique allows the subconscious mind, along with the body and brain, to respond as if this empowered state is real in that moment. By repeatedly engaging in this visualisation, clients begin to influence their neurology to change and strengthened each time they enter this state, both within and outside the therapy room. The more they practise, the more proficient they become, highlighting the significance of repetition in therapeutic success.

For clients with Functional Neurological Disorder, who may struggle with self-doubt and helplessness, ego-strengthening techniques are vital. These methods build confidence and resilience, empowering clients to take an active role in their recovery journey. Therefore, connecting them to their past resources in trance, where they once again get to embody a stronger version of themselves, a version where they have overcome difficult obstacles, and then we encourage our clients to embody these empowering resources in the present and project them into their future. Repetition of these practices enhances their effectiveness, again echoing the principle that the more one practises, the better one gets at it.

CASE STUDY: HYPNOTHERAPY AND FUNCTIONAL NEUROLOGICAL DISORDER

Subject: Sarah, Age 45

Sarah, a 45-year-old woman residing in the beautiful expanses of rural Victoria, had spent a considerable portion of her life hiking and exploring the lush landscapes of the Australian countryside. However, her joy was marred by unexplained perplexing symptoms concerning her mobility that impaired her ability to do what she loved, hiking.

After a prolonged period of misdiagnosis, concern and confusion regarding the causation of her symptoms, she was eventually diagnosed with FND. Sarah experienced intermittent episodes of uncontrollable and indiscriminate mobility issues, ranging from sudden interruptions in her ability to walk normally, to unpredictable leg freezing whereby her legs would not function at all.

What we know about FND is the symptoms may vary significantly. They can fluctuate between severe and normal because the problem is not structural, rather it is due to *how* the brain functions at any given moment. Thus, the brain's networks can shift between maladaptive and normal patterns depending on many psychological factors.

This was the case for Sarah; her symptoms were inconsistent and fluctuated often without warning. On good days, she could stroll through her beloved gardens or go on a bush walk effortlessly. However, on other occasions she would unpredictably find herself struggling to move her legs at all. She experienced these incidences as a 'heavy feeling' in her legs. At these times she felt as though her feet were like heavy concrete, rooted to the ground leaving her completely unable to move them. Her neurologists reassured her that this type of fluctuation in symptom presentation was not unusual for patients with FND. Symptoms often wax and wane, and this is often influenced by environmental stress levels, emotional states, and even physiological changes such as increased sympathetic nervous system arousal in states of heightened anxiety. Hormonal changes or fatigue can also affect symptom expression.

We know that FND involves disruptions in how the brain processes information, particularly within motor and sensory networks and we now see research highlighting the role of neuroplasticity and sensorimotor network activity in FND. What this tells us is that connectivity within these important motor networks can change based on factors such as attention. Clinical hypnotherapists working with clients such as Sarah, can utilise this insight to direct and improve therapeutic outcomes. For instance, if we know that focusing intensely on a symptom like walking difficulty can worsen it and distraction can often lead to improvement, we can build this important principle into the therapy session and the homework tasks. This principle is not unknown to us. It underscores what many practitioners already know: "what you focus on, you strengthen." Therefore, it is crucial to equip our clients with strategies to disrupt patterns of focusing on their symptoms, thereby promoting better symptom management.

After initial discussion with Sarah educating her about the physiology of the mind and body to respond to every thought, we set about creating a process designed to observe her thoughts, monitor her inner chatter and interrupt any unhelpful cognitions. A simple cognitive awareness technique was utilised. As soon as Sarah recognised she was running an unhelpful pattern or focusing on a problem related thought or feeling, she utilised a simple pattern interrupt by taking a breath and redirecting her attention to more solution focused outcomes. In that moment she would imagine that she had already achieved her healthy outcome. As we are all aware one of the most powerful aspects of the subconscious mind is that it is not logical or literal, and it will respond to what Sarah was imagining to be true in that moment as though it was true.

Sarah was acutely interested in learning about how she could effectively rewire the programs she had been running as she set her attention on her intention to be healthy. It became a high priority for Sarah to remember what 'normal' felt like and this is where the hypnotic state became invaluable. We established a very powerful solution state. This was an embodiment of a version of Sarah when the problem no longer existed. Sarah was asked to step into this image many times a day through a self-hypnotic process and she was tasked to interrupt any unhelpful thoughts, feelings or behaviours. She was committed to doing what was required and thus she wholeheartedly embraced her homework tasks.

In the hypnotherapy sessions Sarah embarked on an inward journey with the intention of healing her body. The therapeutic sessions began by fostering a profound state of deep relaxation, and stillness achieved through progressive muscle relaxation and deep diaphragmatic breathing. This enabled Sarah to switch off from the world outside, to connect to her parasympathetic nervous system and retreat inward to find respite from her often worrying and chaotic conscious thoughts.

It was also important for Sarah to challenge all of her unhelpful thoughts surrounding her condition whilst in trance. Metaphorically, these fears were envisioned as clouds passing by in the vast blue sky of her mind, transient, insubstantial, and powerless to do anything but drift away, out of sight, out of mind into the expansive distant blue sky. Through guided imagery, she was encouraged to visualise and embody a life when the FND did not exist, where she was able to move freely, walk in nature and easily pursue her goals.

An important part of her therapy was done using Kinaesthetic Dissociation meticulously woven into the hypnotic sessions. A dissociated technique was safely used during a regression session, employed to uncover the origin of any underlying trauma that may have been precipitating her symptoms. We were able to follow the feeling connected to the current situation all the way back to its origins which involved being sexually abused by her uncle when she was ten years old.

She stated through tears and anger, that she felt powerless. She felt as though her legs were rooted to the ground and she could not run from her abuser. She was directed to focus on her legs and feel the strength in them, to imagine they were so strong they could carry her to safety. When she was completely embodying her strength, she was directed to feel herself running, as fast as she could, running to safety feeling strong and empowered. In the hypnotic state she was given the opportunity to escape her attacker and to tell the adults who would help her. She imagined her uncle going to jail handcuffed by the police. Sarah was able to explore the circumstances of the trauma and safely process the underlying causes that had unknowingly been contributing to her current symptoms.

From a safe dissociated distance, and with the help of the resources she now has that she did not possess when she was ten, she was able to tell her uncle what he had done to her and the impact it had had on her life in so many ways, and that he had no right to do that to her. She said this statement many times getting louder and angrier each time until she felt she did not need to say it further. She stated she was just a little girl he was meant to protect. As her adult empowered self she was able to then take the younger inner child out of danger never to return to that situation again.

By safely revisiting this significant memory, not as a participant but as an observer, Sarah was able to gain understanding of how her past had been affecting her present. She was able to discharge stored emotional energy by connecting to and enacting the resources that she now has as an adult that were not present in her when the trauma occurred. The session allowed her to safely explore these memories, reframing their significance and gently untangling the emotional connections they held.

At the end of the session, Sarah revealed that her symptoms began about two years ago and had progressively worsened since. Her uncle had passed away around that time, and she felt obliged to attend his funeral to support her mother, who remained unaware of her brother's abuse. Sarah stated that she had always avoided family gatherings where her uncle might be present. At the funeral, she experienced a nauseous feeling in her stomach and felt like she wanted to flee, yet her legs did not move. She said that they felt as if they were 'like concrete, rooted to the ground.' The same description she had given about the presenting FND symptoms.

The internal struggle she experienced on the day of the funeral between escaping and supporting her mother had been intense. After the service, she decided to leave saying she wasn't feeling well. The insights that she had gained during the session allowed her to set a new intention, she would tell her mother about the past events. Initially, she said, she thought she was protecting her mother by shielding her from this truth, now after the session she realised, she was inadvertently protecting her uncle, an outcome he did not deserve, and she would no longer do. After the regression session Sarah noticed improvements in her symptoms. The frequency and duration of them was noticeably declining.

A very important question to ask our clients is what was happening around that time when the presenting issue first began. This question had been asked of Sarah, however as her uncle was someone she had consciously shut out of her life, she did not make this connection.

In subsequent session another Visual Kinaesthetic Dissociation technique was utilised in the form of a rewind technique, Once the initiating event had been identified this approach was used to aid in altering how the brain processes and stores the traumatic memory. After rewinding a traumatic memory in a safe dissociated way, we often observe a decrease in symptoms such as anxiety or intrusive thoughts. It is an empowering technique that allows individuals to gain a sense of control over the memory, enabling them to incorporate the experience into their life narrative with diminished distress.

Please refer to chapter 25. Hypnotherapy for PTSD: Reclaiming Control, for more on this technique.

As further sessions progressed, Sarah's focus was on restoring health, her thoughts were solution focused and monitored. Any time old unhelpful thoughts emerged they were quickly allowed to drift away without judgement as she changed her focus to embrace her solution image. She stepped into her future self at the conclusion of all hypnotic sessions and also each day by utilising a self-hypnotic technique. She imagined this future self to have a freedom of uninhibited mobility as she embraced the magnificence of her mind and body's ability to create health. Empowered by this vision, she imagined herself hiking the vast nature trails she so loved and moving through life with newfound health and confidence.

Sarah's symptoms continued to diminish and by session five, approximately two and a half months from her first session, Sarah was walking with ease and had minimal recurrence of past symptoms. She continued to do all the cognitive and self-hypnotic tasks and to take herself out to her healthy future every day. No further sessions were scheduled.

Sarah's journey through hypnotherapy encapsulates a story of resilience, possibility and transformation. It demonstrates that change is possible even when dealing with conditions as challenging as FND. Her case highlights how a blend of therapeutic techniques and self-exploration can foster healing and help to create possibilities rather than limitations.

~

Although research into hypnotherapy for FND is still emerging the evidence to date is encouraging. A recent study explored hypnosis as a potential treatment for FND, highlighting its efficacy in managing various neurological disorders (Connors et al., 2024). Additionally, J. Chen et al., presented at the 2023 International Congress of Movement Disorders where he examined case studies on the use of hypnosis as an adjunctive treatment for FND. The case series involved three adult patients who received virtual hypnotherapy sessions incorporating suggestibility testing, guided metaphors, and individualised post-hypnotic suggestions. The findings demonstrated that all participants experienced significant improvement, with one patient achieving full symptom resolution after a single session and the remaining two achieving substantial symptom reduction after seven sessions. These results suggest that hypnosis may be an effective and accessible adjunctive therapy for FND, particularly for patients responsive to suggestion.

Functional Neurological Disorders challenge our previous understanding of the mind-body relationship, presenting an opportunity to rewrite the old narrative of health and healing. Hypnotherapy, now with its roots in neuroscience and focus on the subconscious, provides a powerful framework for addressing the complex interconnectivity of the psychological, physiological and neurological factors of FND.

Through guided imagery, emotional processing, and the rewiring of neural pathways, hypnotherapy enables clients to reclaim their sense of agency, transforming symptoms from barriers into bridges. As research continues to illuminate the mechanisms of this approach, the potential for hypnotherapy in FND becomes not merely promising, but excitingly profound.

For those living with FND, the message is clear: you are not defined by your symptoms. With the right tools, the brain and body can heal, and you can write a new and more empowering chapter to the story of your life.

Chapter Twenty-Nine

A QUICK WORD ON THE GLOBAL INTEGRATION OF HYPNOTHERAPY IN MEDICAL SETTINGS

As research and evidence supporting hypnotherapy's effectiveness continues to grow, the world is beginning to adopt a new paradigm. Hypnotherapy, once sidelined by conventional medicine, is now boldly entering mainstream healthcare in many diverse ways. This change is being driven by research findings and advancements in neuroscience and technology, which combined are leading to hypnotherapy being recognised as a versatile, evidence-based intervention capable of addressing many complex psychological and physiological challenges. Its growing integration into mainstream medical settings globally marks a significant advancement in holistic healthcare. By acknowledging the intricate mind-body relationship, hypnotherapy is emerging as a vital tool for enhancing patient outcomes.

This shift into mainstream medicine is becoming more visible and in no small part, has been shaped by the dedicated practitioners whose cumulative experiences and outcomes have shone a light on what is possible and in doing so illuminated for the world to see, that which would not stay hidden. These often-outstanding outcomes could no longer be ignored and have stood as a testament to the effectiveness of this wonderfully empowering modality.

As mentioned in previous chapters, hypnosis was historically used in ancient healing rituals before pioneers like Milton Erickson brought it into mainstream practice in the 20th century, effectively shining a light on what was possible when this technique is professionally used to address a myriad of health issues. Now, countries such as Australia, Belgium, Canada, the United States and the United Kingdom have embraced hypnotherapy in healthcare, with more nations following suit.

Here in Australia, we see the Australian Hypnotherapists' Association advocating for the professional recognition of hypnotherapy as an accepted allied health service, and although at the time of this publication government recognition has not yet been achieved, we are observing government bodies such as large public hospitals making up their own mind. Many have funded the treatment of patient sessions for hypnotherapy when other interventions have been ineffective.

The Alfred Hospital in Melbourne, Victoria has a dedicated Functional Gut Clinic where gut-directed hypnotherapy is integrated as part of a multidisciplinary treatment approach involving gastroenterologists, dietitians, psychologists, and hypnotherapists. The clinic holistically manages patients with conditions like irritable bowel syndrome (IBS) and employs hypnotherapists as part of the team providing evidence-based treatment options.

This clinic is currently unique in Australia for its multidisciplinary model combining medical and allied health services for functional gut disorders. It is my hope that very soon we will be seeing many more clinics providing this model of care. The hypnotherapy offered at the Alfred Hospital unit is gut-directed, targeting the brain-gut axis to reduce symptoms and improve digestive health. This pioneering approach is echoed in Canada at the McGill University Health Centre, where hypnotherapy complements traditional treatments emphasising a holistic approach to patient care and recovery.

The Cancer Council of Australia also lists the Australian Hypnotherapists' Association members as recognised providers of support services for individuals affected by cancer. Hypnotherapy is often used as a complementary therapy to help cancer patients manage symptoms and side effects including pain management, reducing anxiety, enhancing relaxation, and lessening nausea related to chemotherapy. This acknowledgement by Cancer Council Australia enhances the credibility of hypnotherapy by endorsing it as a legitimate complementary therapy, thereby validating its role in supporting cancer patients through symptom management and improving overall well-being.

In the ever-evolving landscape of modern healthcare, the transformative power of hypnotherapy is finding its rightful place in mainstream clinics around the globe. From the renowned corridors of the Mayo Clinic in the United States to the trusted NHS in the United Kingdom, hypnotherapy is becoming a beacon of hope for patients seeking relief from chronic pain, anxiety, and a myriad of other conditions.

One of the most well-established applications of hypnotherapy is in pain management. With millions affected by chronic pain worldwide, hypnotherapy offers a non-invasive alternative that addresses both physical and emotional aspects. In Belgium we see that hypnotherapy is part of pain management clinics.

Across the Atlantic to Europe, we find esteemed organisations such as the Charité – Universitätsmedizin Berlin in Germany and the University Hospital Zurich in Switzerland embracing hypnotherapy as a vital component of pain management and psychological support. By using hypnotherapy as part of their integrative medicine services, they aim to provide a holistic approach to patient care that addresses both physical and psychological aspects of health, thus optimising patient outcomes.

Hypnotherapy is also finding itself being well utilised in pre and post-surgical interventions, anaesthesia and dentistry. In mental health, hypnotherapy is proving itself to be transformative, assisting with anxiety, PTSD, and phobias, while complementing cognitive and mindfulness therapies.

While momentum is continuing to grow, challenges such as misconceptions about hypnosis and lack of standardisation persist. Securing government funding remains a hurdle for those who seek to gain government recognition, as does demonstrating hypnotherapy's cost-effectiveness.

Despite the many challenges, the future of hypnotherapy is bright. As it continues to become integrated into many mainstream healthcare facilities, health practitioners are beginning to observe what we hypnotherapists have always known; hypnotherapy is, easily integrated into mainstream medical programs as a complimentary versatile tool for creating holistic healing and growth. Further, in this emerging scientific era, hypnotherapy is continuing to demonstrate that healing often starts from within and it can often be the key to unlocking the mind's vast potential.

Integrating hypnotherapy into medical settings represents a shift in healthcare. As neuroscience and technology continue to evolve, new research is leading to a burgeoning evidence base supporting the efficacy of hypnotherapy. With this comes the potential for further clinical applications in the mainstream arena. This transformative trend sees the fostering of patient autonomy as individuals begin to regain some control over their own mental, physical and emotional well-being on their journey towards healing.

Witnessing the growing acceptance of hypnotherapy in such mainstream medical areas, is encouraging and the future of hypnotherapy looks very strong as more facilities open up to the use of hypnotherapy as an effective modality to manage many conditions. The tide is definitely turning, and with it comes an optimistic future where hypnotherapy is poised to enrich and expand healthcare outcomes, offering comfort and healing in ways once thought unimaginable.

AFTERWORD

As a practitioner of clinical hypnotherapy, I have witnessed this modality creating healing and transformation where none seemed previously possible. I have seen clients who have suffered for years, having consulted countless specialists, yet finding no lasting relief through the conscious mind alone. This is precisely where hypnotherapy comes into its own.

As therapists, we lead the way. Every story of success, every client who finds hope and healing against all odds, adds to a vast body of anecdotal evidence so compelling that mainstream medicine can no longer look away.

Now, with the advancement of technologies such as fMRI, we can literally see what happens in the brain during trance. We can observe the shifts, the changes in neural activity, as the mind quiets its inner critic and reconnects with the body's innate intelligence. In this state, where the conscious chatter falls away, clients can begin to imagine what once felt impossible. They can picture themselves healthy, calm, capable, and that vision begins to take root.

What we know about the brain is that it changes through focus and repetition, and whatever we focus on, we strengthen. This understanding sits at the heart of hypnotherapy where we encourage the deliberate directing of attention toward healing, possibility, and transformation.

We are stepping into a new paradigm, one in which hypnotherapy is no longer seen as fringe or alternative, rather it is now being viewed as an integral part of holistic healthcare. We now see its inclusion in hospitals, dentistry, obstetrics, functional gut clinics, pain management centres, and many other areas of mainstream medicine. As research continues to evolve, a growing body of evidence clearly demonstrates that hypnotherapy is a powerful tool for creating change within both mind and body.

It is an exciting time to be part of this profession. The world is beginning to understand what we, as hypnotherapists, have long known, that the mind has extraordinary power to heal. Change is happening. And one day soon, I believe hypnotherapy will stand alongside other established treatments as a respected and essential therapeutic practice.

As President of the Australian Hypnotherapists Association, I hold a strong vision for the future of hypnotherapy that is both ambitious and inspiring. This vision is not merely a distant hope; it embodies what is not only possible but also achievable through careful integration of the latest scientific discoveries in the fields of neuroscience, epigenetics, bioplasticity, neuroplasticity, and beyond.

As we delve deeper into the intricate workings and remarkable synergy of the body and mind working together in harmony, the evidence from neuroscience continues to gradually merge with a millennia of ancient wisdom and practice. This synergy can lead to extraordinary developments within the realm of hypnotherapy. We stand at the threshold of an exciting evolution in our understanding of the human experience, where the art of hypnotherapy can unlock profound transformation.

We may be witnessing the expansion of human capacity as we step boldly into our divine birthright, that of human potential. This potential is not limited to merely surviving; it encompasses our ability to heal emotionally, physically, and to thrive in all aspects of life. In this journey, we are poised to redefine what it means to be human, embracing our innate capabilities and resilience.

Standing at the precipice of this possibility, we must nurture a belief in our abilities and embrace the feelings and realities of the extraordinary. When we do, we become the creators and directors of our own destinies. Hypnotherapy offers us the tools to harness this transformative power, allowing us to shape our futures in ways we have only begun to imagine.

The future of hypnotherapy is bright, and as we continue to explore and expand this remarkable practice, we will discover new horizons of healing and the potential that awaits us all. Together, we can unlock a world where each person can not only transform their own life but also has the capacity to inspire others to do the same.

I hope this book has inspired you, let us now move forward together, guided by hope, knowledge, and an unwavering belief in the power of the mind.

Welcome to the future of hypnotherapy, a future filled with significant and exciting possibilities.

ABOUT THE AUTHOR

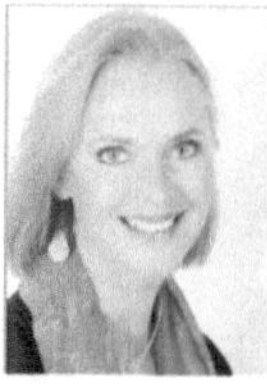

Danielle Aitken is a highly experienced Clinical Hypnotherapist, Counsellor, Registered Nurse and Midwife whose career spans more than four decades across healthcare, mental health, and therapeutic practice. With a strong foundation in evidence-informed medicine and human sciences, including a special interest and further studies in the field of neuroscience, Danielle brings a rare depth of clinical insight to the practice of hypnotherapy.

Her early professional background in nursing and midwifery, including over twenty years working in the demanding field of infertility, genetics and IVF, shaped her deep understanding of trauma, stress, emotional resilience, and the powerful interplay between mind and body. This clinical grounding led her to expand into counselling and ultimately specialise in Clinical Hypnotherapy as a transformational healing modality.

Danielle is the National President of the Australian Hypnotherapists' Association, at the time of publication, where she is a leading advocate for professional excellence, ethical practice, and ongoing education within the field. She is widely recognised for her ability to integrate neuroscience, physiology, and subconscious processes into practical, result-focused therapeutic work.

Through her writing, Danielle bridges the art and science of hypnotherapy, offering both practitioners and clients a clear, credible, and compassionate exploration of how transformational healing occurs.

Danielle's work reflects a lifelong commitment to empowering individuals to access inner resources, restore balance, and create meaningful change.

ALSO BY DANIELLE AITKEN

- **Sarah's Story: Life After IVF**

Project Heart Publishing 2019

- **The Ripples: What Lies Beyond**

Project Heart Publishing, 2020

- **The Health and Happiness Handbook** and
- **The Health and Happiness Handbook Companion Journal**

Project Heart Publishing, 2022

Invited Author Contributor To The Following Anthologies:

- **'Dare to Believe'** in ***Dance in the fire of life***
- ICK.com llc Publishing House, 2019
- **'Are you Listening now?'** in ***The Colours of Me*** MMH Press, 2021
- **Celebrating 365 Days of Gratitude** in ***The Community Book Project 2026***
- Ask And It Is Written Publishing House

Chapter Thirty

BOOKS AND REFERENCES

Akil H, Nestler EJ. The neurobiology of stress: Vulnerability, resilience, and major depression. Proc Natl Acad Sci U S A. 2023 Dec 5;120(49):e2312662120. doi: 10.1073/pnas.2312662120. Epub 2023 Nov 27. PMID: 38011574; PMCID: PMC10710064.

Alladin, A. (2016). Cognitive hypnotherapy for depression: An evidence-based approach. Wiley-Blackwell.

American Psychiatric Association. (2013). Diagnostic and statistical manual of mental disorders (5th ed.). Arlington, VA: American Psychiatric Publishing.

American Society of Clinical Hypnosis. (2025). The neuroscience of hypnosis. ASCH Newsletter. Retrieved 2025, from https://asch.net/newsletter-article/the-neuroscience-of-hypnosis/

Astill Wright L, Barawi K, Kitchiner N, Kitney D, Lewis C, Roberts A, Roberts NP, Simon N, Ariti C, Nussey I, Muss D, Bisson JI. Rewind for Posttraumatic Stress Disorder: A Randomised Controlled Trial. Depress Anxiety. 2023 Oct 12;2023:6279649. doi: 10.1155/2023/6279649. PMID: 40224592; PMCID: PMC11921860.

Barber, J. Hypnosis and Suggestion in the treatment of pain, A clinical Guide Norton Professional Books

Beck, A. T. (1976). Cognitive therapy and the emotional disorders. International Universities Press.

Benson, H., Beary, J. F., & Carol, M. P. (1974). The relaxation response. Psychiatry, 37(1), 37-46.

Brambila-Tapia AJL, Gutiérrez-García MM, Ruiz-Sandoval JL, Vázquez-Vázquez D, Ramírez-Martínez JF, Macias-Islas MÁ, Mireles-Ramírez MA, De-Santos-Fonseca AD, Palomera-Chávez A, Meda-Lara RM. Using hypnoanalysis and guided imagery to identify and manage emotional aspects of multiple sclerosis. Explore (NY). 2022 Jan-Feb;18(1):88-95. doi:10.1016/j.explore.2020.10.002. Epub 2020 Oct 13. PMID: 33132080.

Branden, N. (1994). The six pillars of self-esteem. Bantam.

Bruce Eimer and C. R. Hunter The Art of Hypnotic Regression Therapy: A Clinical Guide

Brown ML, Rojas E, Gouda S. A Mind–Body Approach to Pediatric Pain Management. Children. 2017; 4(6):50. https://doi.org/10.3390/children4060050

Buckner RL, Andrews-Hanna JR, Schacter DL. The brain's default network: anatomy, function, and relevance to disease. Ann N Y Acad Sci. 2008 Mar;1124:1-38. doi: 10.1196/annals.1440.011. PMID: 18400922.

Császár N, Scholkmann F, Bókkon I. Implications on hypnotherapy: Neuroplasticity, epigenetics and pain. Neurosci Biobehav Rev. 2021 Dec;131:755-764. doi: 10.1016/j.neubiorev.2021.10.001. Epub 2021 Oct 5. PMID: 34619172.

J. Chen, J. Waugh, K. Brewer-Mixon, S. Chitnis, D. Morris. Hypnosis as an adjunctive treatment for FND, a case series [abstract]. Mov Disord. 2023; 38 (suppl 1). https://www.mdsabstracts.org/abstract/hypnosis as an adjunctive treatment for fnd a case series/. Accessed October 26, 2025.

Churchill, R. (2002). Regression hypnotherapy: Transcripts of transformation (Vol. 1). Transforming Press.

Connors MH, Quinto L, Deeley Q, Halligan PW, Oakley DA, Kanaan RA. Hypnosis and suggestion as interventions for functional neurological disorder: A systematic review. Gen Hosp Psychiatry. 2024 Jan-Feb;86:92-102. doi: 10.1016/j.genhosppsych.2023.12.006. Epub 2023 Dec 14. PMID: 38154334.

Császár-Nagy N, Bókkon I. Hypnotherapy and IBS: Implicit, long-term stress memory in the ENS? Heliyon. 2022 Dec 30;9(1):e12751. doi: 10.1016/j.heliyon.2022.e12751. PMID: 36685398; PMCID: PMC9849985.

Dahlitz, M. (2017). The psychotherapist's essential guide to the brain. Dahlitz Media.

Dantzer, R., O'Connor, J. C., Freund, G. G., Johnson, R. W., & Kelley, K. W. (2017). Inflammation: The common pathway of stress-related diseases. Frontiers in Human Neuroscience, 11, 316. https://doi.org/10.3389/fnhum.2017.00316

Davidson, A., & Diamond, B. (2001). Autoimmune diseases. In R. M. Mackay & F. S. Rosen (Eds.), Advances in immunology (Vol. 345, pp. 340). N Engl J Med, Vol. 345, No. 5 · August 2, 2001 · Retrieved from : https://www.nejm.org/doi/10.1056/NEJM200108023450506

De Benedittis G. Hypnotic Modulation of Autonomic Nervous System (ANS) Activity. Brain Sci. 2024 Mar 4;14(3):249. doi:10.3390/brainsci14030249. PMID: 38539637; MC10968788.

Del Casale, A., Ferracuti, S., Rapinesi, C., Serata, D., Caltagirone, S. S., Savoja, V., … Girardi, P. (2015). Pain Perception and Hypnosis: Findings From Recent Functional Neuroimaging Studies. International Journal of Clinical and Experimental Hypnosis, 63(2), 144–170. https://doi.org/10.1080/00207144.2015.1002371

Dillworth T, Mendoza ME, Jensen MP. Neurophysiology of pain and hypnosis for chronic pain. Transl Behav Med. 2012 Mar;2(1):65-72. doi: 10.1007/s13142-011-0084-5. PMID: 24073099; PMCID: PMC3717822.

Doidge, N. (2007). The brain that changes itself: Stories of personal triumph from the frontiers of brain science. Penguin Books.

Doidge, N. (2015). Hypnosis, Neuroplasticity, and the Plastic Paradox. American Journal of Clinical Hypnosis, 57(3), 349–354. https://doi.org/10.1080/00029157.2015.985572

Dolcos F, LaBar KS, Cabeza R. Dissociable effects of arousal and valence on prefrontal activity indexing emotional evaluation and subsequent memory: an event-related fMRI study. Neuroimage. 2004 Sep;23(1):64-74. doi: 10.1016/j.neuroimage.2004.05.015. PMID: 15325353.

Domar AD, Rooney KL, Wiegand B, Orav EJ, Alper MM, Berger BM, Nikolovski J. Impact of a group mind/body intervention on pregnancy rates in IVF patients. Fertil Steril. 2011 Jun;95(7):2269-73. doi:10.1016/j.fertnstert.2011.03.046. Epub 2011 Apr 15. PMID: 21496800.

Egner T, Jamieson G, Gruzelier J. Hypnosis decouples cognitive control from conflict monitoring processes of the frontal lobe. Neuroimage. 2005 Oct 1;27(4):969-78. doi: 10.1016/j.neuroimage.2005.05.002. PMID: 15964211.

Elman, D. (1970). Hypnotherapy. Westwood Publishing Company.

Entringer, S., Kumsta, R., Hellhammer, D. H., Wadhwa, P. D., & Wüst, S. (2009). Prenatal exposure to maternal psychosocial stress and HPA axis regulation in young adults. Hormones and Behavior, 55(2), 292-298 PMID: 35180100

Erickson, M. H. (1980). Collected papers of Milton H. Erickson on hypnosis (Vol. IV, E. L. Rossi, Ed.). Irvington Publishers.

Esalen Institute. (n.d.). Animal magnetism. Retrieved April 2025, from https://www.esalen.org/ctr/animal-magnetism/

Facco, E., & Tagliagambe, S. (2021). Learning from the past: From incubation in ancient Egypt and Greece to modern hypnosis. Advances in Social Sciences Research Journal, 8(7), 268–285. https://doi.org/10.14738/assrj.87.10541

Fernandez A, Urwicz L, Vuilleumier P, Berna C. Impact of hypnosis on psychophysiological measures: A scoping literature review. Am J Clin Hypn. 2022 Aug;64(1):36-52. doi: 10.1080/00029157.2021.1873099. PMID: 34748461.

Faymonville ME, Laureys S, Degueldre C, DelFiore G, Luxen A, Franck G, Lamy M, Maquet P. Neural mechanisms of antinociceptive effects of hypnosis. Anesthesiology. 2000 May;92(5):1257-67. doi:10.1097/00000542-200005000-00013. PMID: 10781270.

Faymonville ME, Roediger L, Del Fiore G, Delgueldre C, Phillips C, Lamy M, Luxen A, Maquet P, Laureys S. Increased cerebral functional connectivity underlying the antinociceptive effects of hypnosis. Brain Res Cogn Brain Res. 2003 Jul;17(2):255-62. doi: 10.1016/s0926-6410(03)00113-7. PMID: 12880897.

Faymonville ME, Boly M, Laureys S. Functional neuroanatomy of the hypnotic state. J Physiol Paris. 2006 Jun;99(4-6):463-9. doi: 10.1016/j.jphysparis.2006.03.018. Epub 2006 Jun 5. PMID: 16750615.

Fuhr K, Bender A, Wiegand A, Janouch P, Drujan M, Cyrny B, Schweizer C, Kreifelts B, Nieratschker V, Batra A. Hypnotherapy for agoraphobia-Feasibility and efficacy investigated in a pilot study. Front Psychol. 2023 Aug 10;14:1213792. doi: 10.3389/fpsyg.2023.1213792. PMID: 37637902; PMCID: PMC10448829.

Gay MC, Philippot P, Luminet O. Differential effectiveness of psychological interventions for reducing osteoarthritis pain: a comparison of Erikson [correction of Erickson] hypnosis and Jacobson relaxation. Eur

J Pain. 2002;6(1):1-16. doi: 10.1053/eujp.2001.0263. PMID: 11888223.

Goldberg, A. D., Allis, C. D., & Bernstein, E. (2007). Epigenetics: A landscape takes shape. Cell, 128(4), 635–638. https://doi.org/10.1016/j.cell.2007.02.006

Gruzelier JH. A review of the impact of hypnosis, relaxation, guided imagery and individual differences on aspects of immunity and health. Stress. 2002 Jun;5(2):147-63. doi:10.1080/10253890290027877. PMID: 12186693.

S. M., & Hackett, J. D. (2025). The mind-body connection. In Mind-Body Wellness (pp. 1–17). https://doi.org/10.1007/978-3-031-91611-3_1

Hammond, D. C. (1990). Handbook of hypnotic suggestions and metaphors. Norton & Company.

Hammond, D. C. (2010). Hypnosis in the treatment of anxiety- and stress-related disorders. Expert Review of Neurotherapeutics, 10(2), 263–273. https://doi.org/10.1586/ern.09.140

Häuser, W. (2024). Gut-directed hypnosis and hypnotherapy for irritable bowel syndrome: A mini-review. Frontiers in Psychology, 15, Article 1389911. https://doi.org/10.3389/fpsyg.2024.1389911

Horton-hausknecht, J. R., Mitzdorf, U., & Melchart, D. (2000). The effect of hypnosis therapy on the symptoms and disease activity in Rheumatoid Arthritis. Psychology & Health, 14(6), 1089–1104. https://doi.org/10.1080/08870440008407369

Healthdirect. (2025, May). Phobias. https://www.healthdirect.gov.au/phobias

Heidi Jiang, Matthew P. White, Michael D. Greicius, Lynn C. Waelde, David Spiegel, Brain Activity and Functional Connectivity Associated with Hypnosis, Cerebral Cortex, Volume 27, Issue 8, August 2017, Pages 4083–4093, https://doi.org/10.1093/cercor/bhw220

HGI. (n.d.). The Rewind (de-traumatisation) technique. HGI. Retrieved October 30, 2025, from https://www.hgi.org.uk/discover/mental-health/the-rewind-detraumatisation-technique/

Hou, G., & Li, D. (2014). Possible change process of inflammatory cytokines in the prolonged chronic stress and its ultimate implications for health. The Scientific World Journal, 2014, Article ID 780616, 1–8. https://doi.org/10.1155/2014/780616

Hu P, Lu Y, Pan BX, Zhang WH. New Insights into the Pivotal Role of the Amygdala in Inflammation-Related Depression and Anxiety Disorder. Int J Mol Sci. 2022 Sep 21;23(19):11076. doi: 10.3390/ijms231911076. PMID: 36232376; PMCID: PMC9570160.

Jensen MP, Patterson DR. Hypnotic approaches for chronic pain management: clinical implications of recent research findings. Am Psychol. 2014 Feb-Mar;69(2):167-77. doi: 10.1037/a0035644. PMID: 24547802; PMCID: PMC4465776.

Jensen MP, Jamieson GA, Lutz A, Mazzoni G, McGeown WJ, Santarcangelo EL, Demertzi A, De Pascalis V, Bányai ÉI, Rominger C, Vuilleumier P, Faymonville ME, Terhune DB. New directions in hypnosis research: strategies for advancing the cognitive and clinical neuroscience of hypnosis. Neurosci Conscious. 2017;3(1):nix004. doi: 10.1093/nc/nix004. Epub 2017 Apr 12. PMID: 29034102; PMCID: PMC5635845.

Karlin, R. A., & Orne, M. T. (1997). *Hypnosis and the iatrogenic creation of memory: On the need for a per se exclusion of testimony based on hypnotically influenced recall.* *Cultic Studies Journal, 14*(2), 172–206. https://articles1.icsahome.com/articles/hypnosis-and-the-iatrogenic-creation-of-memor-csj-14-2

Kelly AM, Garavan H. Human functional neuroimaging of brain changes associated with practice. Cereb Cortex. 2005 Aug;15(8):1089-102. doi: 10.1093/cercor/bhi005. Epub 2004 Dec 22. PMID: 15616134.

Kilner JM, Friston KJ, Frith CD. Predictive coding: an account of the mirror neuron system. Cogn Process. 2007 Sep;8(3):159-66. doi: 10.1007/s10339-007-0170-2. Epub 2007 Apr 12. PMID: 17429704; PMCID: PMC2649419.

Kirsch I. Hypnotic enhancement of cognitive-behavioral weight loss treatments--another meta-reanalysis. J Consult Clin Psychol. 1996 Jun;64(3):517-9. doi: 10.1037//0022-006x.64.3.517. PMID: 8698945.

Kohen, D. P., & Olness, K. (2011). Hypnosis and hypnotherapy with children (4th ed.). Routledge/Taylor & Francis Group.

Kuttner, L. (2010). A child in pain: What health professionals can do to help. Crown House Publishing.

Lee HH, Choi YY, Choi MG. The Efficacy of Hypnotherapy in the Treatment of Irritable Bowel Syndrome: A Systematic Review and Meta-analysis. J Neurogastroenterol Motil. 2014 Apr 30;20(2):152-62. doi: 10.5056/jnm.2014.20.2.152. PMID: 24840368; PMCID: PMC4015203.

Landry M, Lifshitz M, Raz A. Brain correlates of hypnosis: A systematic review and meta-analytic exploration. Neurosci Biobehav Rev. 2017 Oct;81(Pt A):75-98. doi: 10.1016/j.neubiorev.2017.02.020. Epub 2017 Feb 24. PMID: 28238944.

Landry M, Raz A. Hypnosis and imaging of the living human brain. Am J Clin Hypn. 2015 Jan;57(3):285-313. doi: 10.1080/00029157.2014.978496. PMID: 25928680.

Lazarus, R. S., & Folkman, S. (1984). Stress, appraisal, and coping. Springer Publishing.

Levitas E, Parmet A, Lunenfeld E, Bentov Y, Burstein E, Friger M, Potashnik G. Impact of hypnosis during embryo transfer on the outcome of in vitro fertilization-embryo transfer: a case-control study. Fertil Steril. 2006 May;85(5):1404-8. doi: 10.1016/j.fertnstert.2005.10.035. Epub 2006 Mar 29. PMID: 16566936.

Liossi C, Hatira P. Clinical hypnosis in the alleviation of procedure-related pain in pediatric oncology patients. Int J Clin Exp Hypn. 2003 Jan;51(1):4-28. doi: 10.1076/iceh.51.1.4.14064. PMID: 12825916.

Liossi C, White P, Hatira P. Randomized clinical trial of local anesthetic versus a combination of local anesthetic with self-hypnosis in the management of pediatric procedure-related pain. Health Psychol. 2006 May;25(3):307-15. doi: 10.1037/0278-6133.25.3.307. PMID: 16719602.

M1 Psychology. (n.d.). Brain waves and hypnosis. Retrieved April 2025, from https://m1psychology.com/brain-waves-and-hypnosis/

Maresca, G., Nocito, V., Lo Buono, V., Latella, D., Di Cara, M., Formica, C., Carnazza, L., Sessa, E., Bramanti, P., & Corallo, F. (2023). Hypnotherapy as a nonpharmacological treatment for the psychological symptoms of multiple sclerosis. Alternatives Therapies in Health and Medicine, 29(4), 266-269. PMID: 35180100.

McGeown WJ, Mazzoni G, Venneri A, Kirsch I. Hypnotic induction decreases anterior default mode activity. Conscious Cogn. 2009 Dec;18(4):848-55. doi: 10.1016/j.concog.2009.09.001. Epub 2009 Sep 25. PMID: 19782614.

McEwen BS. Physiology and neurobiology of stress and adaptation: central role of the brain. Physiol Rev. 2007 Jul;87(3):873-904. doi: 10.1152/physrev.00041.2006. PMID: 17615391.

McClafferty, H. (2018). Mind-Body Medicine in Clinical Practice. (1st ed.). Routledge. https://doi.org/10.4324/9781315157238

Morrison, J. M., & Philips, G. (2001). Analytical hypnotherapy: Theoretical principles (Vol. 1). Crown House Publishing.

Morrison, J. M., & Philips, G. (2002). Analytical hypnotherapy: Practical applications (Vol. 2). Crown House Publishing.

Oakley, D., Halligan, P. Hypnotic suggestion: opportunities for cognitive neuroscience. Nat Rev Neurosci 14, 565–576 (2013). https://doi.org/10.1038/nrn3538

O'Toole SK, Solomon SL, Bergdahl SA. A Meta-Analysis of Hypnotherapeutic Techniques in the Treatment of PTSD Symptoms. J Trauma Stress. 2016 Feb;29(1):97-100. doi: 10.1002/jts.22077. Epub 2016 Feb 8. PMID: 26855228.

Pert, C. (2004). Your body is your subconscious mind. MacMillan Audio

Pessoa, L. (2013). The cognitive-emotional brain: From interactions to integration. MIT Press

Jensen MP, Patterson DR. Hypnotic approaches for chronic pain management: clinical implications of recent research findings. Am Psychol. 2014 Feb-Mar;69(2):167-77. doi: 10.1037/a0035644. PMID: 24547802; PMCID: PMC4465776.

Rainville P, Hofbauer RK, Bushnell MC, Duncan GH, Price DD. Hypnosis modulates activity in brain structures involved in the regulation of consciousness. J Cogn Neurosci. 2002 Aug 15;14(6):887-901. doi: 10.1162/089892902760191117. PMID: 12191456.

Rosendahl J, Alldredge CT, Haddenhorst A. Meta-analytic evidence on the efficacy of hypnosis for mental and somatic health issues: a 20-year perspective. Front Psychol. 2024 Jan 8;14:1330238. doi: 10.3389/fpsyg.2023.1330238. PMID: 38268815; PMCID: PMC10807512.

Rossi, E. L., & Rossi, K. L. (2008). The new neuroscience of psychotherapy, therapeutic hypnosis & rehabilitation: A creative dialogue with our genes. Ernest Rossi.

Rosen, S. (Ed.). (1982). My voice will go with you: The teaching tales of Milton H. Erickson. W.W. Norton & Company.

Rotaru, T. Ștefan, & Rusu, A. (2015). A Meta-Analysis for the Efficacy of Hypnotherapy in Alleviating PTSD Symptoms. International Journal of Clinical and Experimental Hypnosis, 64(1), 116–136. https://doi.org/10.1080/00207144.2015.1099406

Rotimi DE, Singh SK. Implications of lifestyle factors on male reproductive health. JBRA Assist Reprod. 2024 Jun 1;28(2):320-330. doi: 10.5935/1518-0557.20240007. PMID: 38289202; PMCID: PMC11152437.

Sanson, J. (n.d.). Bioplasticity: Hypnosis mind body healing. OA Stories. Retrieved October 29, 2025, from https://www.oastories.org/bioplasticity-hypnosis-summary/

Sauerbrei BA, Pruszynski JA. The brain works at more than 10 bits per second. Nat Neurosci. 2025 Jul;28(7):1365-1366. PMID: 40514587; PMCID: PMC12320479.

Sapolsky, R. M. (2004). Why zebras don't get ulcers: The acclaimed guide to stress, stress-related diseases, and coping. Henry Holt and Company.

Satterfield, J. M. (2013). Mind-Body Medicine: The new science of optimal health [Unabridged audiobook; The Great Courses: Better Living series]. The Great Courses.

Schmidt, H., & Pilat, C. (2023). Effects of meditation on pain intensity, physical function, quality of life, and depression in adults with low back pain: A systematic review with meta-analysis. Complementary Therapies in Medicine, 73, Article 102924. https://doi.org/10.1016/j.ctim.2023.102924

Spiegel, D. (1988). Dissociation and hypnosis in post-traumatic stress disorders. Journal of Traumatic Stress, 1(1), 61-84. https://doi.org/10.1002/jts.2490010104

Spiegel, D. (2013). Tranceformations: Hypnosis in brain and body. Dialogues in Clinical Neuroscience, 15(1), 11–20. https://doi.org/10.1002/da.22046

Spiegel D, Cardena E. New uses of hypnosis in the treatment of post-traumatic stress disorder. J Clin Psychiatry. 1990 Oct;51 Suppl:39-43; discussion 44-6. PMID: 2211565.

Stanford Medicine News Center. (2016, July 28). Study identifies brain areas altered during hypnotic trances. Retrieved April 20, 2025, from https://med.stanford.edu/news/all-news/2016/07/study-identifies-brain-areas-altered-during-hypnotic-trances.html

Technology Networks. (2023, December 17). Caltech scientists have quantified the speed of human thought. Technology Networks. https://www.technologynetworks.com/neuroscience/news/caltech-scientists-have-quantified-the-speed-of-human-thought-394395

Thompson T, Terhune DB, Oram C, Sharangparni J, Rouf R, Solmi M, Veronese N, Stubbs B. The effectiveness of hypnosis for pain relief: A systematic review and meta-analysis of 85 controlled experimental trials. Neurosci Biobehav Rev. 2019 Apr;99:298-310. doi:10.1016/j.neubiorev.2019.02.013. Epub 2019 Feb 18. PMID: 30790634.

Urmston Hypnotherapy. (n.d.). The history of hypnosis. Retrieved April 2025, from https://www.urmstonhypnotherapy.com/the-history-of-hypnosis/

van der Kolk, B. A. (2015). The body keeps the score: Brain, mind, and body in the healing of trauma. Penguin Books.

Vermetten, E., Meijer, L., & van der Hart, O. (n.d.). Hypnosis for PTSD: Evidence based placebo controlled studies. ResearchGate. Retrieved November 1, 2025, from https://www.researchgate.net/publication/281210080_Hypnosis_for_PTSD_Evidence_based_placebo_-controlled_studies

Volgemute K, Vazne Z, Malinauskas R. The benefits of guided imagery on athletic performance: a mixed-methods approach. Front Psychol. 2025 Apr 11;16:1500194. doi: 10.3389/fpsyg.2025.1500194. PMID: 40290535; PMCID: PMC12021890.

Whorwell PJ, Prior A, Colgan SM. Hypnotherapy in severe irritable bowel syndrome: further experience. Gut. 1987 Apr;28(4):423-5. doi: 10.1136/gut.28.4.423. PMID: 3583070; PMCID: PMC1432815.

Wijaya, A., & Trini, I. R. (2023). Effect of hypnotherapy in reducing phobia symptoms. [PDF]. Retrieved from https://pdfs.semanticscholar.org/3f2c/cf086b12979242ec00206d6428e2b5dc6bf1.pdf

Wolf, T. G., Faerber, K. A., Rummel, C., Halsband, U., & Campus, G. (2022). Functional Changes in Brain Activity Using Hypnosis: A Systematic Review. Brain Sciences, 12(1), 108. https://doi.org/10.3390/brainsci12010108

Weiss, B. (1988). Many lives, many masters. Simon & Schuster.

Yapko, M. D. (2013). Trancework: An introduction to the practice of clinical hypnosis. Routledge.

Yehuda R, Hoge CW, McFarlane AC, Vermetten E, Lanius RA, Nievergelt CM, Hobfoll SE, Koenen KC, Neylan TC, Hyman SE. Post-traumatic stress disorder. Nat Rev Dis Primers. 2015 Oct 8;1:15057. doi: 10.1038/nrdp.2015.57. PMID: 27189040.

Zhao, L., & Liu, S.-X. (2022). The application of hypnosis in sports. Frontiers in Psychology, 12, 771162. https://doi.org/10.3389/fpsyg.2021.771162

Zheng, J., & Meister, M. (2025, January 22). The unbearable slowness of being: Why do we live at 10 bits/s? Neuron, 113(2), 192-204. https://doi.org/10.1016/j.neuron.2024.11.008

www.ingramcontent.com/pod-product-compliance
Lightning Source LLC
LaVergne TN
LVHW090315210926
848480LV00001B/250
9780648807896